Psychological Aspects
of Genetic Counselling

Psychological Aspects of Genetic Counselling

Edited by

ALAN E. H. EMERY

The Medical School,
Edinburgh

IAN M. PULLEN

Royal Edinburgh Hospital,
Edinburgh

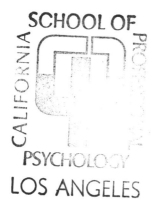

1984   **ACADEMIC PRESS**
(Harcourt, Brace Jovanovich, Publishers)

LONDON · ORLANDO · SAN DIEGO
SAN FRANCISCO · NEW YORK · TORONTO
MONTREAL · SYDNEY · TOKYO · SÃO PAULO

ACADEMIC PRESS INC. (LONDON) LTD.
24–28 Oval Road
London NW1

United States Edition published by
ACADEMIC PRESS INC.
(Harcourt, Brace Jovanovich, Inc.)
Orlando, Florida 32887

British Library Cataloguing in Publication Data

Psychological aspects of genetic counselling.
1. Genetic counselling
I. Emery, Alan E. H.   II. Pullen, Ian
362.1'96042   RB155

ISBN 0-12-238220-X
ISBN 0-12-238222-6 Pbk

LCCCN 83-73148

Photoset by Paston Press, Norwich
Printed in Great Britain by
St Edmundsbury Press, Bury St Edmunds, Suffolk

Contributors

ALDER E., *MRC Reproductive Biology Unit, Centre for Reproductive Biology, 37 Chalmers Street, Edinburgh, UK*

ANTLEY, R. M., *Department of Medical Genetics, Indiana University, PO Box 1367, North Capitol Avenue, Indianapolis, Indiana 46206, USA*

BLUGLASS, K., *St Christopher's Hospice, Park Road, Sydenham, Kent, UK*

BLUMBERG, B., *Department of Pediatrics, The Permanente Medical Group, 2200 O'Farrell Street, San Francisco, California 94115, USA*

BRINGLE, R. G., *Department of Psychology, Indiana University, Indianapolis, Indiana, USA*

DOMINIAN, J., *Department of Psychiatry, Central Middlesex Hospital, Acton Lane, London NW10 7MS, UK*

EMERY, A. E. H., *The Medical School, University of Edinburgh, Edinburgh, UK*

FALEK, A., *Department of Psychiatry, Emory University, Woodruff Memorial Building, PO Box AF, Atlanta, Georgia 30322, USA*

HOLLERBACH, P. E., *The Population Council Center for Policy Studies, One Dag Hammerskjold Plaza, New York 10017, USA*

KINNEY, K. L., *Buchanan Counseling Center, Methodist Hospital of Indiana, Indianapolis, Indiana, USA*

MAGUIRE, P., *Department of Psychiatry, University Hospital of South Manchester (Withington Hospital), West Didsbury, Manchester, M20 8LR, UK*

NORTMAN, D. L., *The Population Council Center for Policy Studies, One Dag Hammerskjold Plaza, New York, New York 10017, USA*

PARRY, R. A., *Royal Edinburgh Hospital, Edinburgh, UK*

PULLEN, I. M., *Royal Edinburgh Hospital, Edinburgh, UK*

RAEBURN, J. A., *University Department of Human Genetics, Western General Hospital, Edinburgh, UK*

ROSENFELD, D. L., *Division of Human Reproduction, Department of Obstetrics, North Shore University Hospital, Manhasset. New York 11030, USA*

WEXLER, N., *National Institute of Neurological and Communicative Disorders, National Institute of Health, Bethesda, Maryland 20205, USA*

Preface

How it comes – let doctors tell

Duncan Gray: Robert Burns

With improvements in living standards and advances in medicine and surgery, infectious diseases and nutritional deficiencies are becoming less common causes of morbidity and mortality. As a result these environmental diseases are gradually being replaced by others which are largely, or even entirely, genetic in causation. The genetic counsellor's role has largely been seen as educational, with the counsellor determining the risks of a particular disorder occurring in a family, and then discussing with the individual couple these risks as well as the various options available to them, should they decide the risks are unacceptably high. However, though this is important, there has been increasing interest recently in the psychological aspects of genetic counselling. Here the emphasis is more on fully appreciating the psychological impact of genetic disease on the individual couple, recognizing the various stages of the coping process, and tailoring counselling accordingly. Only by taking into account the couple's personal background can the various options available be discussed in the most sensitive manner. Thus we are moving away from entirely factually oriented counselling to what Kessler (1979) has called *person-oriented* counselling. In this broader scenario, the demands on the counsellor are much greater but it is only in this way that counselling is likely to be really meaningful and couples helped to make decisions which are the right ones for themselves. There is no place for directive counselling.

The particular qualities which make for a really sensitive and effective counsellor may be largely a reflection of personality and at least partly inherent. However, having said this many of the basic skills of genetic counselling can be acquired by formal training through precept and example (Emery, 1982). The purpose of this book is to provide a guide to some of the more important psychological problems in genetic counselling. It is intended for all those involved in this field including geneticists, genetic associates, paediatricians, obstetricians, hospital physicians, psychiatrists, psychologists, family doctors, social workers and nurses. We hope it might also be useful to medical students and others who wish to know more about current practices in genetic counselling.

After a brief review of the general principles of genetic counselling, there follow discussions of some of the important techniques of counselling particularly in regard to the sequence of responses encountered in emotional crises. Since the occurrence of genetic disease in a family may have serious effects on marital relationships a chapter is devoted specifically to marital pathology. The psychological problems particular to early infant loss, mental and physical handicap, late onset genetic disorders, infertility, sterilization, artificial insemination and prenatal diagnosis are all considered in detail. A final chapter describes how communication skills may be acquired and improved.

Like many other specialities, psychology has its own technical terms which are often somewhat bewildering to the uninitiated. We have attempted to avoid these as far as possible for the benefit of those in other fields. We have also tried to present an essentially practical and common sense approach to the psychological problems of genetic counselling. We do not necessarily agree with everything that each contributor has written, neither do we expect the reader to. However we hope that the book will stimulate thought and discussion about what is a rapidly changing and important subject.

December 1983   *A. E. H. Emery*
                                                                              I. Pullen

Emery, A. E. H. (1982). Postgraduate training in medical genetics. *In* 'Human Genetics – The Unfolding Genome. Proceedings of the VI International Congress of Human Genetics' (B. Bonné-Tamir, *Ed.*), pp. 491–497. Alan Liss, New York.

Kessler, S. (1979). The psychological foundations of genetic counseling. *In* 'Genetic Counseling – Psychological Dimensions' (S. Kessler, *Ed.*), pp. 17–33. Academic Press, New York.

Contents

CONTENTS

1 Introduction – the Principles of Genetic Counselling

ALAN E. H. EMERY

This chapter presents a general introduction to genetic counselling and emphasizes some of the psychological problems involved which are discussed more fully in subsequent chapters. Details of genetic principles as they relate to genetic counselling and risks of recurrence can be found in several excellent texts which deal specifically with these matters (Murphy and Chase, 1975; Stevenson and Davison, 1976; Fuhrmann and Vogel, 1976; Harper, 1981).

Nature of genetic disease

It is useful to consider all disease as being on a spectrum. At one end are those diseases which are very largely environmental in causation and include nutritional deficiencies and infectious diseases. At the other end of the spectrum are the genetic diseases in which environmental factors play no part in aetiology though they may modify the expression of a disorder. These genetic diseases include single gene or unifactorial disorders, which may be inherited as autosomal dominant, autosomal recessive, X-linked dominant or X-linked recessive traits, and cytogenetic disorders in which there is an inherent abnormality of chromosome number or structure. So far some 3000 unifactorial disorders and over 50 cytogenetic disorders have been recognized for which clinically useful catalogues exist (McKusick, 1983; De Grouchy and Turleau, 1977).

Between these extremes of the spectrum lie a group of disorders in which both environmental and genetic factors are believed to be involved in aetiology. These so-called multifactorial disorders include many of the commoner congenital malformations, certain diseases of modern society (coronary artery disease, essential hypertension, diabetes mellitus) and vari-

Psychological Aspects Genetic Counselling

ous psychiatric disorders such as schizophrenia. However, recent research has lead increasingly to the recognition of heterogeneity in many of these disorders and that certain forms may well have a unifactorial basis, for example non-insulin dependent diabetes mellitus of adult onset. The role of genetic factors in multifactorial disorders varies considerably and is much higher in, for example, schizophrenia than in neural tube defects (anencephaly and spina bifida). The greater the role of genetic factors in aetiology, the higher the risks of recurrence in relatives (Skinner, 1983).

The risks of recurrence in relatives are usually high (greater than 1 in 10) in unifactorial disorders, but low (less than 1 in 10) in multifactorial disorders. The risks in unifactorial disorders are determined in a straightforward manner from basic genetic principles. However, in multifactorial disorders such risks are derived empirically (and therefore referred to as *empiric risks*) by actually determining the frequency of occurrence of a disorder among relatives of affected individuals. In cytogenetic disorders the risks depend on the nature of the disorder. In Down's syndrome (mongolism), which is the commonest cytogenetic disorder, most cases are due to an extra chromosome 21 (trisomy-21) and the risks depend on mother's age at conception. A small proportion of Down's syndrome are due to a translocation, where material from chromosome 21 is transferred to another chromosome, and the risks depend on the type of translocation involved and whether it is carried by the mother or the father. Risk figures for unifactorial and some multifactorial disorders as well as for Down's syndrome are given in the Appendix.

Genetic counselling

Genetic counselling is a process of communication between the genetic counsellor and those who seek genetic counselling. The information to be communicated falls roughly into two main areas. Firstly, information about the nature of the disorder: its severity and prognosis and whether or not there is any effective therapy, what the genetic mechanism is that caused the disease and what are the risks of its occurring in relatives. Secondly, information on the available options open to a couple who are found to be at risk of transmitting a genetic disorder. This latter may include discussions of methods of contraception, adoption, prenatal diagnosis and abortion and artificial insemination by donor (AID).

Though essentially an educational process, to be really successful it is important that the counsellor recognize the problems of attempting to communicate information of a personal and delicate nature in a situation where the parents may be grieving over the loss of a child, and which may also be emotionally charged with feelings of guilt and recrimination frequently coupled with a loss of self esteem. The effective communicator in this field is the one who not only recognizes these problems, but can empathize and help a couple transcend them.

Changing patterns in genetic counselling

Over the last twenty years there has been a gradual change in both the mode of referral of individuals for counselling as well as in those seeking genetic counselling (Emery, 1977). Whereas at one time most individuals were referred by hospital physicians, nowadays more are being referred by family doctors, the impetus often coming from couples themselves. Whereas in the past most individuals who sought counselling were from the professional classes and were married, nowadays the social class distribution is the same as in the general population and more individuals now seek counselling before marriage. These changes probably reflect an increasing awareness of the importance of genetic counselling by the medical profession as well as the general population at large. This increasing awareness is no doubt the result of articles in the press, coverage by the news media and more emphasis on genetics in school. These are changes to be encouraged though much still remains to be done in educating both the profession and public about such matters (Childs, 1974).

Coupled with this increasing awareness of genetic disease has also been an increase in what is expected from genetic counselling. All too often in the past some members of the medical profession have tended to view genetic counselling either with nihilism (there is nothing that can be done so why bother with genetic counselling) or with a frankly eugenic philosophy (couples at risk should be *advised* not to have children). However as genetic counselling becomes more informative and helpful and as counsellors are seen to be sensitive to the much wider issues involved in this field, its value is more likely to be recognized and those seeking advice more likely to have their expectations satisfied.

Changing emphasis in genetic counselling

Two or three decades ago genetic counselling was often the province of the scientist, usually as an extension of interests in plant and animal genetics. Understandably this resulted in the emphasis being on genetic mechanisms and risks. Then, largely through the interests of individuals like McKusick, Motulsky, and Clarke Fraser in North America and Carter, Klein, Francois, Böök and Becker in Europe, there was a gradual shift in emphasis to the more medical aspects of genetic disease. This resulted in the recognition of the widespread occurrence of genetic heterogeneity: that clinically similar disorders could be inherited differently and have different prognoses. Subsequent developments led to the redefining of recurrence risks in many genetic disorders.

Recently the emphasis has begun to change again from what Kessler (1979) has referred to as *content-oriented* counselling to *person-oriented* counselling with more emphasis on the psychological aspects of genetic counselling. This change of emphasis has resulted from the recognition of a number of important factors. Firstly, that information about genetic disease is rarely emotionally neutral and often has profound psychological effects. Secondly, these effects may have long-term consequences and extend throughout the family to other relatives. Thirdly, and perhaps most importantly, has been the realization that couples given genetic counselling may opt for a course of action which may be at variance with what the counsellor might have regarded as reasonable. There is often a gap between the counsellor's expectations and the actual consequences of counselling. For example in a two-year follow-up study of 200 consecutive couples seen in a genetic counselling clinic, over a third of those who were told they were at high risk of having a child with a serious genetic disease were undeterred and actually planned further pregnancies (Emery *et al.*, 1979). In the past such behaviour has often been regarded as 'irresponsible', a failure on the part of the counsellor and an indictment of counselling in general. But when the couples in this study were carefully questioned their reasons for planning further children were often very understandable.

For example, further pregnancies were planned in some cases because, after seeing the effects of a disorder in a previous child or in one of the parents, it was not considered sufficiently serious (congenital cataract, congenital deafness, peroneal muscular atrophy), or prenatal diagnosis was available (Sandhoff's disease, X-linked mental retardation) and yet in other cases the parents planned further pregnancies because if a subsequent child were affected it would not survive (renal agenesis) or if it survived it would succumb within a year or so (Werdnig–Hoffmann disease). There was also a small but lamentable group of couples who had no living children and dearly wanted a family at whatever cost.

Thus a course of action which might seem irresponsible to one person may be eminently reasonable to another. In a free society this choice is the individual's prerogative provided it is made in the full knowledge of all the facts and appreciation of the possible consequences. Since the counsellor's role is to help couples reach decisions which are the best for themselves genetic counselling should always be non-directive (Anon, 1982).

The genetic counsellor's role

With this change of emphasis the genetic counsellor is now seen to have two major roles: not only to communicate factual information but also, armed with an appreciation of the psychological aspects of the problem, to help couples in their decision making. It is no longer sufficient to be conversant merely with the genetic and medical aspects of a problem. It is also important to be fully aware and appreciative of the psychological effects on the individual. Only in this way can the counsellor empathize and thereby be a more effective communicator. These latter skills are much more difficult to acquire. Formal training (Emery, 1982) through precept and example is important but the qualities which make for a really sensitive and effective counsellor may be largely a reflection of personality and at least partly inherent.

Nevertheless the genetic and medical aspects should not be underestimated. It is a *sine qua non* that the first step in genetic counselling is the establishment of a precise diagnosis especially because of the possibility of genetic heterogeneity. The counsellor also needs to be as conversant, as is reasonably possible, with all the important medical aspects of a genetic problem if counselling is to be at all meaningful.

Problems in counselling

Because of the intense emotional stress often engendered by genetic disease, genetic counselling should only be given in a relaxed and quiet atmosphere where couples can be encouraged to ask questions and express their feelings. Only in this way is it possible to explore a couple's attitudes to a genetic disorder and their interpretation of its implications.

As a prelude to genetic counselling it is important to divine a couple's educational and social background, their religious attitudes and, if possible, something of their marital relationships if information is to be presented most effectively and sensitively.

Having initially established a precise diagnosis, the genetics of the condition and family details, how much further the counsellor should proceed depends on how far a couple will welcome and benefit from more information at the time. Immediately after the loss of an affected infant or immediately after the diagnosis of a serious genetic disorder has been made is not the time for detailed and extensive discussions because the parents are unlikely to be either receptive or comprehending. To know precisely when and how much information to impart during the grieving period requires considerable skill and understanding. The various stages of the so-called 'coping process' have to be recognized and subsequent counselling tailored accordingly (Falek, 1977).

Having decided the time is right to proceed further with counselling, the relevant medical and genetic details of the disorder and the risks of recurrence can be presented. With regard to the medical details, information should be available on such matters as age at onset, progression, complications, the ultimate prognosis and possibilities for effective treatment. Much has been written on the concept of 'burden' in genetic disease by which is meant the psychological, social and, to a lesser degree, financial problems associated with such diseases. A disorder in which the burden is great but short lived (for example a child born with a lethal congenital malformation) may be far more acceptable, even if the risk of recurrence is high, than a disorder where the burden is moderate but protracted (such as a child with slowly progressive and disabling muscular dystrophy).

Unlike the clinician concerned with management and who must therefore maintain a positive and optimistic approach throughout, the genetic counsellor has to present an accurate picture even if depressing and disturbing if the parents are to make a reasoned decision about future children. In this regard the counsellor is therefore often seen as the 'harbinger of woe'. It is questionable whether it is right to encourage parents in the hope that any future affected children might be treatable when at present there is little likelihood of this. Such discussions of treatment in any future affected children require considerable sensitivity when the parents already have an affected child. In fact it is not uncommon for the genetic counsellor to find himself in this dilemma and therefore to have to temper his remarks very carefully.

In most cases it is doubtful if genetic mechanisms and recurrence risks need be discussed in much detail. The actual interpretation of risk is in any event very subjective (Pearn, 1973). Certainly a pedantic obsession with risk figures by the counsellor may completely obscure the real issues and detract from effective communication on more important matters. Nevertheless risks form a useful basis for further discussion and in general terms can be a significant factor in influencing parents' decision making (Carter et al., 1971).

Turning to the options available to a couple who decide they could not accept an affected child, prenatal diagnosis has been a major development and has removed much of the uncertainty in genetic counselling (Table 1.1.). Here developments are taking place so rapidly that it would not be unreasonable to hold out this option in some cases where at present this is not yet possible (Galjaard, 1980). Again however care is necessary for it would seem unreasonable to have a couple delay planning a pregnancy in the hope of a reliable prenatal diagnostic test becoming available in the near future when at present there seems little likelihood of this. In the waiting period there is also

Table 1.1 *Main indications for prenatal diagnosis*

---

(1) Cytogenetic abnormalities
. mainly Down's syndrome with a previously affected child or maternal age
>35–40·

(2) Inborn errors of metabolism
. over 60 can now be diagnosed *in utero*
. most are rare recessive disorders

(3) Fetal sexing
. X-linked disorders which cannot yet be diagnosed *in utero* (e.g. Duchenne
muscular dystrophy)

(4) Congenital abnormalities
. mainly neural tube defects with a previously affected child or raised maternal
serum alphafetoprotein
. some others can be diagnosed by fetoscopy or ultrasonography

---

always the danger of an unplanned pregnancy, and in any event an exaggerated concern with this possibility could well lead to serious marital problems. Both these eventualities could be prevented by careful and detailed discussions of contraceptive methods at an early stage in counselling.

When parents decide that they could not accept having an affected child and prenatal diagnosis is either not possible or, for whatever reason not acceptable, then other options have to be considered. Contraception in this context requires expert advice because the results of failure will be far more devastating when there is the risk of a severely affected child than when it is practised for social or economic reasons. Further, the very deep fear of having an affected child may well generate serious psycho-sexual problems which can often be prevented only by resort to definitive contraceptive methods such as sterilization. However abstinence may be the only acceptable alternative to some couples and these cases require sympathetic understanding and perhaps a discussion of other forms of sexual relief. The latter may be particularly important in any event in those genetic disorders which lead to physical disability in one of the parents (e.g. adult forms of muscular dystrophy). However not all counsellors will feel competent or confident to discuss such very personal matters in which case they should refer a couple to someone who is.

At one time adoption was often an option which could be encouraged by the genetic counsellor but in the last few years this has become increasingly difficult. This is partly because some adoption agencies have become reluctant to place children in families where a parent may have a disabling disorder, but mainly because fewer children are now available for adoption. Before even raising this option it is therefore advisable for the counsellor to determine beforehand whether, in a particular case, this is likely to be a realistic possibility. Otherwise there can be considerable frustration and disappointment.

Finally AID might be offered where it is known that both parents carry the same *rare* recessive gene or the father has an autosomal dominant disorder or carries a chromosome translocation which in the unbalanced state is likely to result in an affected child, e.g. Down's syndrome. However, the success rate, even in expert hands, is not always high and several inseminations may be necessary before success is achieved (Richardson, 1975). Again considerable frustration can result unless a couple are warned about these problems beforehand. Understandably many couples also find this an unacceptable option for personal and aesthetic reasons and if the counsellor senses this the subject should of course not be pursued.

Conclusions

There are essentially three aspects to genetic counselling. The scientific aspect is concerned with genetic mechanisms and risks of recurrence. It is perhaps the least important. The medical aspect is concerned with diagnosis and the resolution of genetic heterogeneity and is an essential first step in counselling but it should be viewed only as a preliminary to a consideration of the wider issues. The psychological aspect of genetic counselling is concerned with understanding and appreciating the psychological effects of genetic disease so that more effective communication is possible. Couples are thereby helped to make decisions which are the best ones for themselves in their particular circumstances and which may not necessarily be those which the counsellor would have made. However, having witnessed so much suffering and unhappiness caused by genetic disease, it is understandable that many genetic counsellors, despite themselves, may harbour the deep-seated wish that when faced with the dilemma some couples would be wise to exercise caution . . .

> Past sorrows, let us moderately lament them;
> For those to come, seek wisely to prevent them.
>   John Webster's *The Duchess of Malfi*, 1616

References

Anon (1982). Directive counselling. *Lancet* ii, 368–369.
Carter, C. O., Roberts, J. A. F., Evans, K. A. and Buck, A. R. (1971). Genetic clinic – a follow-up. *Lancet* i, 281–285.

Childs, B. (1974). A place for genetics in health education, and vice versa. *Amer. J. Hum. Genet.* **26**, 120–135.

De Grouchy, J. and Turleau, C. (1977). 'Clinical Atlas of Human Chromosomes'. John Wiley & Sons, New York.

Emery, A. E. H. (1977). Changing patterns in a genetic counseling clinic. *In* 'Genetic Counseling' (H. A. Lubs and F. de la Cruz, Eds), pp. 113–120. Raven Press, New York.

Emery, A. E. H. (1982). Post-graduate training in medical genetics. *In* 'Human Genetics – The Unfolding Genome. Proceedings of the VI International Congress of Human Genetics' (B. Bonné-Tamir, Ed.), pp. 491–497. Alan Liss, New York.

Emery, A. E. H. (1983). 'Elements of Medical Genetics'. 6th ed. Churchill Livingstone, Edinburgh and London.

Emery, A. E. H., Raeburn, J. A., Skinner, R., Holloway, S. and Lewis, P. (1979). Prospective study of genetic counselling. *Br. Med. J.* **1**, 1253–1256.

Falek, A. (1977). Use of the coping process to achieve psychological homeostasis in genetic counseling. *In* 'Genetic Counseling' (H. A. Lubs and F. de la Cruz, Eds), pp. 179–188. Raven Press, New York.

Fuhrmann, W. and Vogel, F. (1976). 'Genetic Counselling'. 2nd ed. Springer-Verlag, Berlin.

Galjaard, H. (1980). 'Genetic Metabolic Diseases – Early Diagnosis and Prenatal Analysis'. Elsevier/North-Holland, Amsterdam.

Harper, P. S. (1981). 'Practical Genetic Counselling'. John Wright, Bristol.

Kessler, S. (1979). The psychological foundations of genetic counseling. *In* 'Genetic Counseling: Psychological Dimensions' (S. Kessler, Ed.), pp. 17–33. Academic Press, New York.

McKusick, V. A. (1983). 'Mendelian Inheritance in Man'. 6th ed. Johns Hopkins Press, Baltimore.

Murphy, E. A. and Chase, G. A. (1975). 'Principles of Genetic Counselling'. Year Book Medical Publ., Chicago.

Pearn, J. H. (1973). Patients' subjective interpretation of risks offered in genetic counselling. *J. Med. Genet.* **10**, 129–134.

Richardson, D. W. (1975). Artificial insemination in the human. *In* 'Modern Trends in Human Genetics' (A. E. H. Emery, Ed.), Vol. II, pp. 404–448. Butterworths, London.

Skinner, R. (1983). Genetic counselling. *In* 'Principles & Practice of Medical Genetics' (A. E. H. Emery and D. Rimoin, Eds), Vol. 2, pp. 1427–1436. Churchill-Livingstone, Edinburgh.

Stevenson, A. C. and Davison, B. C. C. (1976). 'Genetic Counselling', 2nd ed. Heinemann, London.

2 Basic Counselling Techniques

RICHARD PARRY

Introduction

Throughout this chapter, I shall refer to 'the doctor' and 'the patient'. These words may not be strictly appropriate. The counsellor may not be *medically* qualified. However, the patient often depends upon him in the same way and this is constructive. Furthermore, in genetic counselling, people who come for advice may be perfectly healthy, so that the word 'patient' is inappropriate. However, these terms are convenient for purposes of discussion and are hallowed by medical tradition.

Many doctors are uneasy about counselling. It does not seem to be the province of respectable specialities. Doctors are busy people. Their time must not be wasted on extravagances which could be managed perfectly well by others. What if they say the wrong thing? May not that have serious consequences? Anyway, what is counselling? Surely no more than explanation and reassurance, making suggestions and giving advice? The sort of thing that doctors do all the time.

It is certainly true that some doctors offer many suggestions and much advice in the belief that they are counselling. Unfortunately, as they are often aware, their efforts do not always seem to be very successful. Counselling itself is not an examinable subject, and little attention is paid to it by any of the Royal Colleges – even the Royal College of Psychiatrists!

In the early stages of medical training, the prospective doctor develops a technique, often based on trial and error, of history-taking. He learns gradually that certain questions lead most patients to give certain replies. He learns to avoid the questions which give answers of the wrong sort, even though they may be very revealing. Consequently, his technique may become stereotyped and errors ingrained. The faulty techniques acquired may eventually relegate the patient to the role of a 'yes-man' to the medical mogul. He is rewarded with approval if his answers dovetail into the

Psychological Aspects Genetic Counselling

inquisitor's preconceived ideas. If they do not, he is labelled as a poor informant or a contradictory and unreliable historian. Volumes of crucial information are lost.

Some believe that the whole problem will soon be solved by electronics. A user-friendly computer, equipped with a voice analyser, will take the place of human fallibility. It will ask only the right questions. All investigations will be undertaken by technicians, guided by other computers. The conclusions will then be printed out on a television screen.

Until this dreadful day arrives, those doctors who yearn for them try to avoid contact with patients, particularly when they have distressing news to impart. They leave the matter to the general practitioner, or to the nursing staff ('. . . just have a word with Sister. She'll give you a cup of tea . . .').

But real medicine can never abandon the humanity which is the basis of its existence. Counselling is one of its primary skills. Counselling helps to provide information and to bring comfort. Patients *want* to talk to *doctors*, and to be talked to by doctors. *They nearly always feel better for having done so.* This is one of the great mysteries of medicine. At the end of what, to the doctor, may have seemed a fruitless interview, patients often say, 'Thank you so much for your help. I feel very much better, just for having spoken to you'. In seeking to counsel about counselling, we aim to make the practice of interviewing as fruitful for the doctor as it is beneficial to the patient.

As in many branches of medicine, such as operative surgery, counselling is a *practical* skill. It is learned by doing. Inevitably, mistakes may be made. Even sophisticated, experienced senior physicians sometimes make mistakes. Fortunately, they can nearly always be corrected. If they are recognized and acknowledged, they are rarely repeated. The doctor must be willing to accept that he is fallible. All doctors are fallible: it takes a little courage to acknowledge the fact. Sometimes mistakes can be turned to the patient's advantage. How rarely can such a thing be said about other iatrogenic misfortunes!

It is preferable that a doctor should acquire the elements of counselling skills early in his career. He will never know everything because every patient gives, seeks, requires and receives something different. The ultimate aim is to elicit the maximum of significant information in the most lucid and comprehensive way; to evaluate that information and to learn how to follow it through.

When facility in exercising counselling skills has been acquired, it will be found to be surprisingly economical in medical time. But the facility takes time to acquire and needs practice. Perhaps it is strange that a house surgeon, who takes more than an hour to perform his first appendectomy, should expect to acquire a corresponding skill without practice. Yet many do. It is expected of them by their teachers – some of whom have never acquired it themselves.

The doctor

In hospital practice (and sometimes in general practice, too) patients often complain that they 'never see the same doctor twice'. Profusion of specialists and division of chores means that there is at least a grain of truth in this complaint. It certainly 'feels' very true to the patients who make it.

In complex situations, particularly those in which stress and delicacy are involved, it seems desirable that there should be one person, not necessarily of senior status, whom the patient can identify as 'the doctor'. 'The doctor' provides a consistent link between hospital and the patient, keeps abreast of the progress of the 'case' and will be present when important decisions are made. It may be he who undertakes the first enquiries, conducts a general physical examination and initiates preliminary investigations. If he is junior, he will consult frequently with his senior colleagues, but to the patient, he is 'my doctor', and will be held in special regard. This is to the advantage of everyone.

The doctor's task appears easy. In fact, it is extremely arduous. It is to give the patient his complete and objective attention. Gentleness, humanity and sensitivity will make his work easier, whether he is eliciting an accurate initial history, formulating a plan of campaign or assisting the patient to accept the outcome – whatever it is.

Thus, the doctor brings a new dimension to the 'case'. It is one of great subtlety.

Procedure

To the patient, out-patient clinics are often frightening, bustling places. Sometimes they seem to have as many rooms and corridors leading from them as in a French farce. Nurses in their confusing grades of uniform, people in white coats of varying length and cut, mingle with shabby and smart civilians (the consultants), all of them going, very fast, somewhere else.

Doctors often use the excuse of being busy to hide the fact that they are rather unpunctual people. Even when he has been ushered into their presence, the patient may have to wait, feeling like an unwelcome intruder. It is necessary for the doctor to be *alone* with his patient if he is to do his job properly. It is true that some doctors – especially those who are rather vulnerable and unsure of themselves, those who do not know what is expected of them or what they are supposed to do – are alarmed at the prospect of being alone with a patient. Doctors such as these welcome the 'rational' excuse of being busy. However, in a matter as subtle and delicate as genetic counselling, it is better for the doctor to learn to substitute such fears with concern for his patient. So, when the patient arrives at the appointed time, his doctor is ready to greet him. He gives his bleep to his secretary, tells his friends that he is not to be disturbed and ensures that a plain nurse is allotted to him. Then he sits down with the patient.

This simple act is itself alarming to some doctors. They prefer to sit on the other side of the desk away from, rather than with the patient. The idea of sitting *with* a patient suggests an intimacy which is slightly disconcerting. The doctor feels exposed. But although the desk separates the doctor from the patient, it also separates the patient from the doctor. The physical barrier symbolizes a psychological one. There may be many barriers to be overcome. It would be better to indicate, without the use of words, that they are not impenetrable. The present author prefers the desk to be on one side of the room. He and the patient sit away from it, in armchairs, placed at roughly 90 degrees to each other. He can observe the patient throughout the interview. The patient can look away if he wishes to do so.

The doctor and the patient are sitting together. What happens next? What do they talk about? In counselling, it is often a good idea to begin with whatever is uppermost in the patient's mind. We might make a reasonable guess that the first thing with which a patient is preoccupied is the very fact of attending a genetic counselling clinic. Probably he has been concerned with the idea ever since it was raised: perhaps to a degree to which even sleep itself was becoming difficult or impossible. Doctors, wakening on the morning of their 'new patient' days, rarely give thought to the fact that what is routine for them, may be totally absorbing and rather frightening to the patient, who wakened some hours earlier.

So the doctor might ask the question, 'How did you feel about coming here?' (note that he does *not* say 'Were you frightened of coming here?' The reason will be discussed shortly). Having put the question, the doctor must *wait* for the reply. It may take several moments for the patient to gather his thoughts. Sometimes, his mind goes completely blank. At others, he finds himself struggling with powerful emotion. By his relaxed attention, the doctor imparts reassurance to the patient. He does not need to use words. Silently, he seems to say, 'Take your time. I know it's difficult'.

Eventually a reply will come. It is not necessary to comment on it. Some doctors say, 'Lots of people feel like that' or 'Perhaps it won't be as bad as you think'. The first reply invokes a statistic. Statistics apply only to groups of people, not to individuals, so they are superfluous. The second predicts a judgement, but it is one for the patient to make, not the doctor. Perhaps it will be *worse* than he thinks! Whilst such comments are meant kindly, they are of little value and are best avoided.

The act of answering the question, 'How do you feel about coming here?', may have an unexpected consequence. The disagreeable feeling is dissipated.

When feelings have been expressed, they often fade away. The ground is thus cleared for the detailed history, to which the doctor may now proceed.

The framing of questions

At this point, it is appropriate to remind the reader of some of the technical points about the framing of questions. There are two basic types of question: the 'leading', and the 'open-ended'. Leading questions usually require only a brief reply, such as, 'yes', 'no', '27', 'Friday', or 'measles'. Leading questions are sometimes used as devices to obtain speedy factual information. In some respects, they appear to bring precision to the interview. Thus, leading questions are used when the patient is asked his name, his address, his date of birth, his occupation and the name of his general practitioner.

But the apparent precision may be specious. The patient is given little flexibility in which to frame his reply. Consequently, significant and relevant information may be missed or delayed. The leading question, 'Do you become breathless when climbing stairs?' may seem to be irrelevant to patients who live in bungalows. If the patient fails to realize what the question is *supposed* to mean, he may, knowing that doctors are busy men, answer questions too literally. This problem is solved by phrasing the question in the open-ended form: 'What sort of things make you short of breath?' The answer requires a little thought, and a sentence or two in reply. It provides no guidance as to the direction in which the patient should turn his thoughts. It was for this reason that the preliminary question, 'How do you feel about coming here?' was cast in the open-ended form. Although it was probable that the patient was anxious at the prospect, it is best not to *lead* him into saying so. In medicine, it is a useful aphorism that there is nothing so obvious that it can be predicted with certainty. Occasionally, the patient's response is something other than that of anxious anticipation. Some experienced physicians have considerable difficulty in changing their life-long habit of asking leading questions: a useful formula is to form them around the words 'How do you feel about?' or 'Tell me about'.

When asked about attending a specialist clinic, some patients will reveal elaborate fantasies, based on the alleged experiences of acquaintances, friends or relatives, sensational and largely fictional journalism, or half digested information obtained from the radio or television. The doctor need not be in too much of a hurry to correct such misapprehensions. First, he should pay attention. From time to time, he can put himself into the patient's shoes with the comment, 'It must have been very frightening to think that such a thing might be done to you'.

When asking questions, the doctor should always use short sentences and simple words. Positive questions are to be preferred to negative ones. 'It is by no means far from infrequently that the absence of tubercle bacilli is not invariably detected'. [Quoted in 'The Seven Sins of Medicine' by Richard Asher, *Lancet*, **2**: 358–360 (1949)]. Only one question should be asked at a time and multiple questions should be avoided. Occasionally, the doctor will find that he has phrased a question badly, or that somehow he has asked the 'wrong' question. He should let it stand and, as always, listen carefully to the reply. Sometimes the patient answers the 'right' question. Sometimes his reply to the 'wrong' question gives unexpected and revealing information.

Content of the discussion

It may be helpful to the patient to identify the matters which are to be discussed. This is so especially when they are to be delicate or intimate. The doctor may say, 'I want to ask you about the sexual side of your marriage'. Obviously, such things must not be avoided, although they are sometimes as embarrassing to the doctor as they are to the patient. However, like naked-ness, the doctor will become accustomed to such matters. When he becomes less embarrassed, so will the patient.

The patient's reaction to intimate questions may be a general increase of tension. Occasionally, the doctor will feel that he has touched upon a very delicate area indeed: one about which there may be much more to be said. The doctor may succeed in reducing the tension by speaking directly about it. He may say, 'It's a bit embarrassing to talk about such things'. The patient may admit or deny any embarrassment. The doctor should observe: he need add no more.

A few patients, asked about sexual matters, dispute whether such questions are 'really necessary'. This reaction is a direct expression of what is known as 'resistance'. The word explains the mechanism. The doctor should avoid a direct answer, taking it for granted that his questions are all 'really necessary'. Instead, he may reply, 'It sounds as though you are reluctant to talk about such things'. As always, he waits for the reply. It may not be immediately forthcoming and he should not try to hurry it. However, if the patient is very silent, it is sometimes helpful to repeat the comment.

Obvious questions about sexual matters include frequency of intercourse, ejaculation, climax and fidelity. The replies given will usually suggest further questions. Sometimes, replies are made in a tone of voice which itself requires elucidation. For example, an interview may proceed as follows:

DOCTOR (announcing the theme): 'I want to ask you about the sexual side of your marriage'.

PATIENT (perceptibly uncomfortable): 'Of course. All part of the job'.

DOCTOR (speaking directly of the emotional reaction in order to reduce tension): 'You find it a bit embarrassing?'

PATIENT (giving a laugh which isn't a laugh): 'Not at all'.

DOCTOR (gently persistent): 'People often find sexual matters embarrassing at first'.

PATIENT (capitulating): 'I suppose so'.

DOCTOR (reverting to the specific topic): 'About sexual intercourse'.

PATIENT (slightly too quickly): 'Yes?'

DOCTOR (feeling that he must tread firmly but gently. He does not ask a question): 'Frequency varies a lot in different couples'.

PATIENT (babbling): 'I suppose it does'.

DOCTOR (very gently): 'Would you give me an idea of the frequency in your own case?'

PATIENT (warily): '. . . er . . . It varies'.

DOCTOR (persisting): 'Would you give me an idea?'

PATIENT (apologetically): '. . . er . . . Not very often'. (As if it were an explanation). 'We are both very busy. Perhaps about . . . say . . . er . . . fortnightly?'

DOCTOR (noticing the patient has asked a question, although she does not really put it into words. She is saying, 'Is that satisfactory?' The doctor does not answer. In particular, he is careful to avoid critical comments such as, 'Is that all?' or 'As often as that?' Instead, he tries to bring precision to the reply by using a leading question): 'When was the last time?'

PATIENT (very long pause).

DOCTOR (intuitively): 'It sounds as though it was more than a fortnight ago'.

PATIENT (defensively): 'Well, as I say, we're both very busy. It probably was more than a fortnight. Say a month'.

DOCTOR (careful not to let the matter descend into a sort of auction): 'You're making me think that it was a very long time ago'.

PATIENT (perhaps relieved to be able to get it off her chest): 'Well certainly it isn't very often. That's true'.

DOCTOR (intuitive again): 'Something you miss?'

PATIENT (starting to cry): 'Well you can't help . . . after all . . . you have your feelings . . .'

It is thus becoming apparent that there is a serious sexual difficulty between the patient and her husband. The reader may be wondering what all this has to do with genetic counselling. It is this. Marital problems occur in medicine in all sorts of disguises: in the fertility clinic, the gynaecological, endocrine and genito-urinary clinics as well as in the psychiatric clinic. They may certainly reveal themselves in the genetic counselling clinic. In the present case, there is now little point in pursuing *genetic* counselling. It will first be necessary to deal with the interpersonal problems. By careful attentive questioning, the doctor has saved much valuable time.

Compare this with the outcome if the doctor confines himself to a series of leading questions:

DOCTOR (busily): 'No sexual problems?'*
PATIENT (very hurriedly): 'No'.
DOCTOR (relieved to be finished with it. He uses two questions 'to save time'): 'Frequency and fidelity OK? (Telephone rings) 'Yes, Yes, Yes, Yes. OK Bye. . . . Sorry about that. Frequency and fidelity OK?'
PATIENT (too late now to go back): 'Yes'.
DOCTOR: 'We'll have to do some tests . . .'
PATIENT 'Yes' (a mixture of relief at getting away with it and disappointment, because she knows that the opportunity has been lost).

Note how leading questions have dramatically reduced the time devoted to the interview. Imagine how much time will now be wasted on fruitless investigations.

The good news and the bad

Doctors have little difficulty in conveying what they presume to be 'good news'. However, the word 'good' involves a judgement, and in counselling the doctor should avoid judgements of any kind. It *should*, of course, be 'good news' to both partners if they can be assured that there is every reason to suppose that their children will be genetically normal. But there are some cases when it would be preferable if the news were 'bad'. Such cases occur when, for example, the marriage is unstable or unsatisfactory. Some people, although happy about their marriage, have mixed feelings about bringing up children. They themselves may be rather immature and dependent, emotionally unprepared or possibly too self-centred to undertake the obligations of parenthood. To such people, 'good' news may be bad, and 'bad' news good.

Such occasions are infrequent, but when they occur, the doctor will often sense that his 'good' news is received without the enthusiasm which he had expected. He may ask the patient about his response. The reply may be rather half-hearted, such as 'I'm very pleased, of course, but . . .'. The doctor must ask for elucidation of the 'of course, but'.

'Bad' news hurts the patient. Doctors do not like hurting patients and some try to avoid such disagreeable tasks. They hope that bad news will diffuse through to the patient by some sort of psychological osmosis. The consequence is that some patients never hear the outcome of investigations and live

---

* Technically, this is a forcing negative leading question. Any reply will be ambiguous. The patient's predictable reply was 'no'. This means, literally, 'yes'. It is almost impossible for the patient to answer the question in a way which indicates that she has a sexual problem. Hence it is a 'forcing' question.

with the optimistic, but unjustified assurance that 'they would have told me if there had been anything wrong . . .'.

When the news is bad, many doctors try to comfort the patient with a conventional cliché which is supposed to act as an anodyne. 'Think of all the people who are worse off than you' they say. Such remarks are of no value and may even be regarded as offensive. If bad news has to be given, sympathy alone is required. Gratuitous comments should be avoided.

It takes time to give bad news. This, more than any other, is an occasion when the doctor must ensure that he has time to spare. He should not blurt out the bad tidings, call for a cup of tea and excuse himself because there are other things to be done.

It is without question that doctors are busy, but their time must be used to the patient's best advantage. When he has been given bad news, it is to the patient's best advantage that the doctor should sit with him. The patient may cry. The doctor should let him do so. The patient may search for an explanation. He may find something to condemn in himself – perhaps a minor peccadillo which dates back for many years. The doctor should not try to 'reassure'. He may ask, 'Has this been a worry to you all these years?'

The patient may be angry and try to blame others: his marital partner, or other doctors who have treated him. The doctor should allow the patient to express these feelings, too. He need not rush to anyone's rescue. If the patient is angry, he should be allowed to say so. He should be encouraged to express his feelings, whatever they are, to whomsoever they are addressed.

The expression of emotions usually has a beneficial effect, and they should be released as soon as possible. Delay leads to wasteful preoccupation, and may turn unresolved grief into destructive illness.

Denial

So far, we have assumed that patients accept bad news immediately and without question. This is not always so. Before they accept, many go through a phase of 'denial'.

In its technical use, this word is much stronger than in everyday speech. The patient seems to say, 'It is simply not true. The news is *not* bad'.

As a consequence of denial, the patient may feel that, for example, it is just a bad dream: that he will waken to find that all is well. Some say that they feel 'numb'. Some insist that there has been a mistake, and accuse the physician for example of muddling blood samples. They doubt the conclusions, question the data and refer to new treatments which have been evolved in other countries. Sometimes, they will say bleakly that they do not believe it.

The function of 'denial' is to protect the patient from the painful truth. It *denies* reality and is, therefore, *illogical*. Consequently, it cannot be overcome by logic. It is not amenable to argument. The physician should not allow himself to become involved in an argument. Neither should he be offended. He must appreciate that, at the moment, the news is too painful to be accepted. Sympathy and compassion is required. The physician should be wary of any tendency to become angry, resentful or rejecting. He may say, 'What I have said must sadden you deeply.'

If the facts are *clear*, he should resist all pressures for a second opinion. It would be inhuman to do so, holding out hope when there is none.

Denial ultimately gives way to *acceptance*. When acceptance is completed, the patient moves into a third, constructive stage of *restitution*. 'If that is the way things are' he seems to say, 'we must do something about it'. He starts to take a fresh interest in life and makes constructive plans for the future. His mood lightens perceptibly.

Ambiguous news

Despite their protests to the contrary, patients often invest doctors with an aura of omniscience. As a result, when the news is ambiguous, they may find it difficult to comprehend. They cannot be given hope, neither need they be given despair. The patients are very puzzled and sometimes they protest 'You must surely know best, doctor'. Other patients seize on the fact that an optimistic outcome is possible and speak as though it is assured. The doctor may have difficulty in convincing them that it is uncertain.

The decision

Whether the news is good, bad or ambiguous, a decision must be made. Especially when it is ambiguous, the patient will look for help in making it. If there is a considerable element of chance, the doctor will be placed in the uncomfortable position of helping the patient to take a rather inhuman gamble.

Although the patient will have the last word, there is no reason why the physician should not share the *moral* responsibility. (Obviously, he cannot accept the legal responsibility for the decision).

In *sharing* the responsibility, the physician may find it difficult not to *influence* the patient. When the situation is ambiguous, the patient will often prefer the path which he would have taken had it been favourable. The patient is helped by the knowledge that he has the *support* of his physician. However, if the outcome is unsatisfactory, the physician may feel a double burden.

When more than one person is concerned – husband and wife, for example – it may be useful if they are always seen together. It is common for patients to mis-report medical comments and advice, and the consequences may be undesirable. Errors are minimized when the people concerned are seen together. We have emphasized that it is important to pay attention to what the patient says. It is also important to attend to what they say to each other. When he conducts joint or multiple interviews, the physician should listen to each person in turn. He should discourage one from 'talking over' the other. If a husband wishes to disagree with his wife, he should be asked to listen carefully to what she has to say, first. When she is finished, he can have his turn. Then the wife must listen carefully. She may not interrupt until her husband has finished.

Patience is a great virtue, easier for some than for others, and easier to exercise with some patients than with others. It is the cornerstone of successful counselling. Important clues will be missed or overlooked if the doctor is not prepared to be patient with his patient. Patience is the most delicate, the most subtle and the most rewarding of the medical arts.

Further discussion of these, and other aspects of counselling, will be found in the author's book, 'Basic Psychotherapy' (Second Edition, 1983), Churchill Livingstone, Edinburgh and London.

3 Sequential Aspects of Coping and Other Issues in Decision Making in Genetic Counseling

ARTHUR FALEK

Introduction

The essence of genetic counseling is the counselor's ability to transmit genetic information about an inherited disorder of concern to the counselee(s) so that it will be incorporated into decision making. In addition to basic genetic probabilities, the counselor should also help evaluate alternative options stemming from the multiple concerns raised by the diagnosis. These include identification of various support services for the patient as well as other members of the family. A realistic appraisal of all information needs to be provided and discussed so that the counselee is aware of all possible choices.

In contrast to the idealized counselor goals of genetic counseling (Fraser, 1974; Falek, 1977; Antley, 1979; Kessler, 1979) are the contradictory reports from different outcome studies of follow-up reproduction, particularly among those individuals concerned with recurrence of high risk genetic disorders. These findings suggest a need either to improve communication methodology or revise the counselor's expectations of counseling.

Some years ago, for a conference on genetic counseling, we reported the importance of employing the coping process as a means by which counselors could impart necessary information for understanding and decision making as well as to achieve psychological homeostasis. The theme of that report was on counselor recognition of the various stages of the coping process as they relate to the comprehension of new genetic information, as well as its incorporation at the emotional levels (Falek, 1977).

The psychological aspects of genetic counseling were first emphasized by Kallmann (1956) a generation ago in his presidential address to the American

Society of Human Genetics. He stated that there was need to combine the information portion of genetic counseling with personalized guidance based on sound psychological principles. Our report on coping aspects of genetic counseling was also derived from an earlier publication (Falek and Britton, 1974) on the more general phenomenon of stress and coping in which grief and/or bereavement reactions were a special type.

The coping responses of individuals under stress were considered as phenotypic expressions of psychological mechanisms attempting to re-establish the dynamic steady state. The sequence of responses commonly observed in individuals under stress is: (1) shock and denial; (2) anxiety; (3) anger and/or guilt; and (4) depression as stages that individuals experience in the process of achieving (5) psychological homeostasis. These stages are essential elements of the coping response to a stressful event. The new information must be received and incorporated on both cognitive and emotional levels before any behavioral adjustments can take place.

Assessing the effects of counseling

At the time of our initial report (1977) there were relatively few papers measuring 'outcome' in this area. At present, with a marked increase in genetic counseling programs throughout the United States, United Kingdom, Canada and other parts of the world, there are a series of reports on the impact of genetic counseling on those who seek such help (see above).

It is of interest that the apparent measure of success of genetic counseling is reduction of reproduction in those at high risk for recurrence of a genetic disorder, in particular those with severe clinical consequences. Emphasis on reduction of public health costs by amniocentesis and abortion of affected offspring as the significant measures of success in genetic counseling could provide for the rebirth of some of the negative aspects of the now defunct eugenics movement once directed towards 'race improvement'.

In contrast to reduction of public health costs, it would seem appropriate that the major goal of genetic counseling should be improved quality of life for the families that seek such help (Twiss, 1979). One result of the latter concept will be when the role of the counselor as a family adviser is in opposition to the position he may have as a public health official. The counselor must be aware of the role he is assuming in a particular genetic counseling situation (Childress and Casebeer, 1979). Futhermore, those who train genetic counselors need to identify such differences and discuss them in order to help clarify genetic counseling strategies in a variety of circumstances. This should be introduced into training programs before the unsavory history of the eugenics movement is repeated once again, but this time utilizing more precise scientific procedures.

In this regard it is important that a recent statistical analysis of the effect of genetic counseling on 200 couples (Evers-Kiebooms and van den Berghe, 1979) showed that past reproductive experience and parental desire for children explained far more of the variance in reproductive outcome than did such variables as reproductive risk, burden of the genetic diorder, education background, or socio-economic status. Furthermore, the observation that reproductive risk, as provided in genetic counseling, was not a major determinant of post-counseling reproduction was also reported by Sorenson and colleagues (1980). They also found that genetic counseling did not affect the reproductive intentions of a large majority of women who had initially stated their intentions prior to counseling. In a review of nine follow-up studies of the impact of genetic counseling, Evers-Kiebooms and van den Berghe (1979) indicated widely different findings among investigators as to counselee understanding and recall of recurrence risks, as well as the influence of genetic counseling on counselee decisions about family planning. They emphasized the need for adequately designed and methodologically sound genetic counseling projects, as valid conclusions could not be drawn from many of the programs reported up to 1979.

Hsia (1977) indicated that strategies for the appraisal of genetic counseling needed to differentiate between *what* information was conveyed and the *way* in which information was conveyed. He emphasized that there was a need to know how acquired genetic knowledge influenced parental attitudes as well as their capacity to cope with their problems. Based on the Evers-Kiebooms and van den Berghe (1979) suggestions, a controlled retrospective follow-up of the effects of genetic counseling on parental reproduction after the birth of a child with Down's syndrome was recently reported by Oetting and Steele (1982). Twenty-three couples who had received genetic counseling after the birth of the affected child were matched with twenty-three couples who had not received such genetic counseling. It was found that there were no significant differences between counseled and non-counseled couples in their knowledge of general genetics, recurrence risk for Down's syndrome, initiation or intention to initiate subsequent pregnancies or use of pre-natal diagnosis. In fact, only three of the eighteen couples who initiated at least one more pregnancy after the birth of their Down's syndrome child, used prenatal diagnosis by amniocentesis to determine whether they had another affected child. A similar finding was reported by Oakley and colleagues (1979) who noted that neither professional, nor lay education, nor even cost, were the primary reasons for the apparent rejection of prenatal diagnosis for Down's syndrome by the majority of older mothers. The authors indicated that until this kind of behavior was understood, genetic counseling with prenatal diagnosis would only have a limited impact on reducing the incidence of Down's syndrome. As emphasized by Lippman-Hand and Fraser (1979), more important than diagnosis, prognosis and risks were the counselees' perceptions of the factual information. The psychological state of the parents under stress – how they perceived the factual information – seemed more important for their decision than what actually the facts were.

The coping process

What is known is that all individuals coming for genetic counseling are under stress. The psychological sequence of events that evolves prior to decision making is the coping response.

Shock and denial

The initial response of an individual faced with a stressful situation which could disrupt the psychological equilibrium is to attempt to maintain the status quo by *denial*. The first response in the sequence, therefore, is shock and disbelief. Psychological mechanisms attempt to maintain the integrity of the personality simply by denying the stressful situation. Since the individual does not acknowledge the stress at either the cognitive or emotional level, he is not motivated at this point to initiate the change necessary to adjust to the new reality.

Denial may take many forms. The individual temporarily may appear stunned or dazed, refuse to accept the information given, insist there is some mistake, not comprehend what has been said, and so on. Genetic counselors have reported evidence of this by describing responses to information on diagnosis, mode of transmission, or recurrence risk as 'it is God's will', 'God wouldn't do that to us', as well as the pragmatic response 'give it to me straight, I can handle it'. Frequently the patient firmly entrenched in denial is considered to be the 'good client' because he 'accepts it so well'. To those unaware of the psychological manifestations of the coping response, such an individual may seem to be very mature in his attitude and his handling of the situation.

What needs to be understood is that the denial mechanisms act as 'shock absorbers' to reduce the impact of the sudden trauma and prepare the individual for cognitive acceptance of the situation. The duration of the denial period depends upon the individual and the circumstances, but may be quite short-lived. In some instances this 'shock phase' may be so brief as to be missed by an ordinary clinical observation. No matter how brief the time of denial the counselor must be aware that the patient, at this stage, is only able to absorb little, if any, new information. This may be the reason that recall of genetic counseling information is limited when given at the same session where the diagnosis is presented.

Anxiety

The second stage of the coping process is when the individual becomes more aware of the reality and attempts to deal with the new situation at the intellectual level. It is at this stage that various manifestations of *anxiety* are demonstrated. These include nervousness, overactivity, irritability, headaches, fatigue, insomnia, loss of appetite, and somatic complaints. The individual perceives the change produced by the stressful situation but, since he has not yet adjusted psychologically to his new reality, he experiences fear, and may become panic stricken. His anxiety is a response to the fear of the perceived change in his psychological equilibrium. However, he has not yet experienced a change in psychological equilibrium at the emotional level. The stressful event has been incorporated at the intellectual level only.

During this period of anxiety, the individual initiates intellectual activities directed towards re-establishing equilibrium. In his search for alternatives he may, for example, seek new information which will help him to understand, or perhaps to undo, the predicament. It is at this point with counselees who are not at extreme levels of anxiety that the counselor will be able to present the genetic information and initiate discussion of alternative courses of action. Knowledge of genetic disorder in an immediate relative may affect and alter the response to everyday, as well as unique, stressful events.

There are studies directed towards further understanding the structure and process of coping and these need to be applied to the exploration of the psychological aspects of genetic counseling. Such studies could help in assessing the range of anxiety within which there is acceptance and incorporation of new information. Once there is acceptance, is there an optimum speed of processing information for short- and long-term storage as a basis for help in decision making? Furthermore, is there a specific range of anxiety levels within which cognition occurs, and what are the variations in that range between individuals?

A 'Ways of Coping Checklist' is available which attempts to separate information-favored-problem-focused coping from emotion-focused coping (Folkman and Lazarus, 1980). As indicated by the latter authors, there is an overlap between the two areas. In genetic counseling while the emphasis is on the effect of the emotion-focused aspects of coping, counselees need to be provided with measures to assess specific areas of problem-focused coping. Not only has medical science, including genetic counseling, been unaware of the importance of the coping response as a basis for decision making, but Pearlin and Schooler (1978) note that the social sciences have also given limited attention to the coping process.

In order to evaluate the coping responses of genetic counselees an assessment must be made of the psychological resources and the personality characteristics that people themselves draw upon in order to withstand the threats of the events imposed upon them by their circumstances. The 'Ways of Coping Checklist' is one attempt to measure such factors.

Janis and Mann (1977) believe that, to produce a successful emotional impact, it is necessary to interfere with the person's spontaneous effort to ward off his awareness of the sign of impending danger. Where necessary, unwelcome findings need to be conveyed to the counselee to provide a realistic picture of the disturbing events. Such information has to be presented without provoking either extreme panic or adverse avoidance reactions such as defensive indifference and denial.

The counselee's responses are related to ego involvement based on how the individual perceives the threat as relevant to his personal goals, decisions, and social commitments, as well as his basic personality characteristics, including his chronic level of anxiety. While it is the counselor's task to propose realistic alternatives, as well as to elicit others from the client, the need is to be able to recognize and provide appropriate support for those with high anxiety.

For those with high anxiety it is suggested (Kallmann, 1956) that the best method is to offer a low key presentation of the 'threatening' information. For those with relatively low anxiety, the best responses were found with strong appeal data. The counselor must recognize that during this stage the highly anxious counselee will block all information. It must be remembered that in spite of understanding and appreciating the need for change, the counselee, in fact, still hopes for a magical return of the old *status quo*. The extremely anxious person remains hypervigilant and, if not provided with a low key version, will be unable to process the information and proceed to the subsequent stages of the coping process.

Anger and guilt

With the inability to accept emotionally the new information, attempts at re–adjustment will result in failure. As intellectual manoeuvres to disregard the new information prove unsuccessful, frustration is experienced and the individual may become bitter and hostile. Therefore, there is need through-out the counseling sessions for the counselor to maintain the individual's level of self-esteem, not only for the affected individual but also in high risk carriers. Constant denial and long–term avoidance of real problems tends to be maladaptive and results in *anger* and *frustration*. It should be recognized that such resolutely bitter, hostile or angry individuals are frustrated persons who are unable to proceed through this particular stage of the coping reaction. Under such circumstances they cannot process new information and foster the appropriate actions. This results in angry individuals who see their misfortunes as acts of a cruel and uncaring world. In such a state, a person may be hostile to those around, including friends, relatives, and medical personnel, without a rational basis for their antagonism.

Anger may also be directed inwardly, resulting in feelings of *guilt*. Both the guilt-ridden and the angry individual is attempting to resolve conflicts and frustrations by seeking an agent responsible for his stress. An experienced counselor may be able to channel the guilt and redirect the anger. At times, however, the counselor is seen as an *agent provacateur* who is only multiplying the counselee's problems. In such instances, it is best for the counselor to withdraw, but leave the door open for the counselee to return at a later date.

Strategies to deal with coping and adaptation as part of the decision-making process include counselor sensitivities to such issues as assessment, motivation, information seeking and utilization, contingency planning, rehearsal, trial actions, feedback, social influences, channeling priorities, preparation, and prescription. For the genetic counselor there is not only the need to identify and assess the success of various coping strategies by adults, but also by children in order to deal with maladaptive actions within families who seek help.

Depression

The change from guilt or anger to *depression* is the signal to the counselor that the individual is entering the next phase of the coping reaction. The depression results from the repeated frustration of attempts to resolve the problem. The individual is faced with the emotional burden of the trauma and becomes depressed. The genetic counselor has to be sensitive to the emotional presentation, as well as the cognitive linkages that may be identified during a genetic counseling session. The depressed individual appears sad, withdrawn, and may exhibit a lack of interest in his environment and usual activities. As with denial, anxiety, and anger, depression is a normal phase of the coping process necessary for eventual re-adjustment.

Psychological homeostasis

Registering the alteration of psychological equilibrium ushers in the beginning of adaptive change. As the client recognizes that his old patterns will not resolve the current problem, he begins trying new ones. The role of the counselor is to support the client in his attempts to try alternatives. At this stage, the counselee is most receptive to new ideas. The counselor has to be cautious, in order to avoid the client incorporating the counselor's points of view in his decisions without evaluation.

This is a critical time in the genetic counseling process. If the client can, with the counselor's support, formulate and carry through his own program of decisions, then it is a learning experience which he can apply to other aspects of his current problem, as well as to other situations. If, on the other hand, he is only following the prescription of the counselor, the experience will not be an educational one. There will be no reinforcement or carry over, even if the prescription works out to his advantage.

As new patterns of behavior are learned, repeated, and found to be successful, they will become reinforced and established as normal responses to the problem at hand. A counselor should expect cycling between the coping phases, and for the coping process to continue to occur after an initial approach to psychological homeostasis.

To cope effectively the individual must be able to make decisions using the newly incorporated information by initiating appropriate problem solving. The aim of the genetic counselor should be to encourage the individual to evaluate alternative courses of action with regard to outcome, in order to implement the most appropriate one (Janis and Mann, 1977; Janis, 1974). The counselor should be aware of the social support and health agencies which could be helpful to families with specific genetic disorders. Where possible, cohesive family structures should be identified and used, although it must be remembered that there are family members who, rather than help, may enhance the stress and inhibit coping (Folkman, Schaefer and Lazarus, 1980). To achieve a consistent pattern of change it is most important for the counselor to support and reinforce appropriate actions by the client.

The coping process, as presented here, is an attempt to explain the psychophysiological functions that regulate the control of emotional distress and enhance information processing. All contributors to the field of stress and coping, whether they emphasize the psychodynamic or cognitive aspects of the coping process, indicate the great importance of maintaining the counselee's self-esteem. What cognitive psychologists indicate, in addition, is that it is possible to develop and provide strategies to the counselees in anticipation of problems that lie ahead. Those with self-esteem will employ the agreed upon strategies in order to deal with the specific problems that have previously been discussed.

Only a limited number of sessions will be required for those not at risk of developing or transmitting the disorder under investigation. For the majority of such individuals, all that is necessary will be a restatement of the facts at a later date. However, even for persons apparently with minimal involvement (e.g. an identified clinically unaffected, heterozygous carrier of a gene for a rare, autosomal recessive trait), as well as for those with realistic concerns, the initial behavioral change after the genetic information is presented and discussed will often only approximate the necessary behavior for the establishment of the new psychological steady state. The individual temporarily may experience frustration as he tries out his new behavior patterns, and will revert to some earlier phase in the coping process. He may repeat the entire coping sequence many times or fluctuate between two dominant phases. At present, it is believed that the characteristic pattern the individual displays will depend upon his previous coping experience, genetic make-up, and the complexity of the problem for which counseling has been sought. This includes both the pattern of responses and the length of time required to re-establish the steady state.

According to this coping hypothesis, it seems that, as the individual makes closer and closer approximations to the behavior necessary for the re-establishment of the steady state, the intensity and the length of time spent in each of the coping phases will diminish. In addition to the ego involvement and the anxiety level of the counselee, social support could help facilitate the individual's coping efforts.

As the coping sequence is repeated with diminishing intensity, the individual will be eased into a new psychological equilibrium, which can be maintained because gradually it has been incorporated at both the intellectual and emotional levels. This may be seen as the protective function of the steady state mechanism on the psychological system for it allows the individual gradually to establish new equilibria as he constantly re-adjusts to the stresses introduced by the information given to him in genetic counseling sessions.

Decision making

At present, the stated goal of genetic counseling is the transmission of scientific information about the particular genetic disorder of concern to the counselee, while the implied goal is the reduction of reproduction in counselees who have a high probability (≥ 10 per cent) of having an affected child. As noted previously, while some counselors have expected such information to dissuade high risk family members from planned reproduction, a number of studies of reproductive outcome after genetic counseling did not find the expected results. If genetic counseling is non-directive, then counselors should expect varied responses from counselees. In part, this may be a consequence of the ambiguity or uncertainty of the risk information provided in genetic counseling. In such cases inferences assume critical importance (Folkman, Schaefer and Lazarus, 1980). While for some, inferences as to the meaning of the given odds may reduce their ambiguity, for others it may encourage distortion of the threatening information. Thus, a 50 per cent chance of a recurrence risk may appear remarkably high for some, while others will see that risk only as a 50 per cent chance of having a normal child.

Although ambiguity or uncertainty about outcome and the desire for a normal child plays a role in the reproductive choices of some parents who have a child with a high recurrence risk genetic disorder, it is certainly not the whole story. This is indicated by the observation that when probability can be made a certainty (as is reported above in the study of the frequency of use of prenatal diagnosis to detect a second Down's syndrome child) very few parents still opted for amniocentesis in a future pregnancy (Oetting and Steele, 1982).

In the United States, the constant attention by the mass media given to anti-abortionists and their denouncements (based in large measure on fundamentalist religious beliefs and to some degree on moral human rights convictions) may even influence some who would seek an abortion for an abnormal fetus, and must have an impact on some high risk parents. The negative focus of these presentations challenges prospective parents, as well as society, as to their moral values and self-esteem if the affected fetus is aborted. For those unprepared for this challenge to their humanity and self-esteem, this must make the decision whether to abort or accept responsibility for the birth of a seriously affected child a very difficult one.

While there is the assumption that it should be possible accurately to predict the actions of individuals by measurement of their attitudes about possible future events, this may not be so for such a basic emotionally charged biological desire as reproduction. For example, there is frequently a discrepancy between an individual's attitudes prior to the onset of a disorder, and his behavior after the event has occurred (Antonovsky, 1972). As indicated in an article about the cognitive biases that stem from reliance on judgemental heuristics (Tversky and Kahneman, 1974), for judged probabilities to be considered adequate or rational, internal consistency is not enough. They found that the judgements must be compatible with the entire web of beliefs held by the individual, and that such information was hard to obtain even with our most sophisticated measures.

Further analysis of decision-making by these authors (Tversky and Kahneman, 1981) clarified their thoughts about how individuals evaluated the relative attractiveness of the different options available. They found that the appeal of the options varied when the same problem was framed in different ways. It was their opinion that a change in perspective would lead the decision-maker to reconsider the previously rejected, original preferences even in the absence of objective standards. This did not imply preference reversal nor was it necessarily irrational. It was proposed that the decision-maker should focus on future experiences to frame potential outcomes in order to select the best one. This suggests that additional time is required in genetic counseling sessions to provide counselors with objective information about affected individuals in a variety of settings. Such information, perhaps, would be transmitted most successfully in role playing sessions or by providing the counselee with the opportunity to visit an individual affected with the particular genetic disorder and his family. The counselees could then return for objective discussions about the disorder and its many potential effects (economic, medical and social). While such programs would add to the complexity of genetic counseling, it would, hopefully, provide the counselees with more useful and meaningful information about the disorder in question.

Would the finding of the failure of mothers of a Down's syndrome child to request amniocentesis in subsequent pregnancies refute this suggestion? It may well be that amniocentesis was not desired in these cases because there are only minor differences to be seen between infants and very young children with Down's syndrome and normal babies. It is only when Down's infants mature that the differences become more pronounced. This may be one reason why some of the women in the study of parental reproduction following the birth of a Down's syndrome child (Oetting and Steele, 1982), both in the test and control groups, did not request amniocentesis. On the other hand, it may be that amniocentesis for those women implied a high risk of abortion which was not acceptable to those who agreed to participate in the investigation. However, prevention of reproduction was also not an acceptable outcome. If these women were deciding to have a child in the full understanding of the possible consequences (one of which was the birth of a second Down's syndrome child), then we consider such an outcome was not a failure in genetic counseling. From a strictly cost–benefit analysis, however, each such pregnancy that went to term without amniocentesis and abortion of the Down's fetus would be designated as a failure of genetic counseling. Private or public funds would be required for infant stimulation, vocational rehabilitation, sheltered workshops, halfway houses and medical facilities to provide lifetime support. It would have been of interest to learn whether other contraceptive options were discussed in the genetic counseling sessions, and, if so, with what result.

Direct and non-directive counseling

A more recent suggestion is the need to return to a directive approach for genetic counseling using decision analysis (Pauker and Pauker, 1977). Computer focused decision analysis has been reported in other medical specialties as a basis for determining the optimal treatment strategy when expert opinions are widely discrepant (Ransohoff and Feinstein, 1976; Weinstein and Findeberg, 1980). Problems with this type of decision procedure include the difficulties of identifying and incorporating all the relevant issues for analysis

(Brett, 1981; Kassirer and Pauker, 1981). This is particularly the case when the differences in the probabilities indicate a 'toss up' decision for either of two procedures. Other concerns are the ethical issues resulting from such an approach, including how much weight should be given to whether those making the decision (experts, parents, etc.) have a high or low tolerance for undesirable consequences. The report on a computer based decision program in genetic counseling (Pauker and Pauker, 1977) was directed towards parental decisions about amniocentesis and abortion in Down's syndrome, meningomyelocele and Duchenne muscular dystrophy. The analyses include parents' knowledge about the disorder as well as measures to quantify their attitudes to amniocentesis, abortion, and having an affected child. It is expected that these objective studies will help the parents make a rational decision about prenatal diagnosis after weighing the best outcome (an unaffected child) against the relative costs or burdens of other outcomes including therapeutic abortion, spontaneous abortion or birth of an affected child.

There is no indication that this directive approach to genetic counseling has been tested. The question is whether such an approach would have changed the attitude to amniocentesis of mothers with an increased risk of a Down's syndrome child. Psychostatistical data on the complexity of outcome for all forms of probability-derived decision-making would suggest little, if any, change in the reported results with the directive approach. What seems evident from the Tversky and Kahneman (1981) report is that decision-making is altered by changes in the individual's perceptions of the problem and shifts in the reference point when the same problem is framed in a different way.

Conclusions

The function of the genetic counselor is to provide information about the disorder in question and its recurrence risks at a time in the coping process when the individual is able to accept the new information and incorporate it into his belief system. How the newly incorporated information is employed in decision-making, in particular about procreation, is evidently more complex, and should not be used as the basis for evaluation of genetic counseling.

Analysis of the coping process provided in this chapter suggests that the most propitious time to assess an individual's cognitive functions during stress is during the stage of anxiety. Finally, there is concern about the divergent conscious and unconscious biases of genetic counselors who report that they provide non-directive counseling, and then indicate as failure a lack of decline in reproduction of those at high risk for serious genetic disorders.

References

Antley, R. M. (1979). The genetic counselor as facilitator of the counselee's decision process. *Birth Defects* **15**, 137–168.

Antonovsky, A. (1972). The image of four diseases held by the urban Jewish population of Israel. *J. Chron. Dis.* **25**, 375–384.

Brett, A. S. (1981). Hidden ethical issues in clinical decision analysis. *N. E. J. Med.* **305**, 1150–1152.

Childress, J. F. and Casebeer, K. (1979). Public policy issues in genetic counseling. *Birth Defects* **15**, 279–290.

Coelho, G. V., Hamburg, D. A. and Adams, J. E. (1974). 'Coping and Adaptation'. Basic Books, New York.

Evers-Kiebooms, G. and van den Berghe, H. (1979). Impact of genetic counseling: a review of published follow-up studies. *Clin. Genet.* **15**, 465–474.

Falek, A. and Britton, S. (1974). Phases in coping: the hypothesis and its implications. *Soc. Biol.* **21**, 1–7.

Falek, A. (1977). Use of the coping process to achieve psychological homeostasis in Genetic Conditions. *In* 'Genetic Counseling' (H. A. Lubs and F. de la Cruz, Eds), pp. 179–191. Raven Press, New York.

Folkman, S. and Lazarus, R. S. (1980). An analysis of coping in a middle-aged community sample. *J. Health Soc. Behavior* **21**, 219–239.

Folkman, S., Schaefer, C. and Lazarus, R. S. (1980). Cognitive processes as mediators of stress and coping. *In* 'Stress and Cognition' (V. Hamilton and D. M. Warburton, Eds), pp. 265–298. John Wiley, New York.

Fraser, F. C. (1974). Genetic counseling. *Am. J. Hum. Genet.* **26**, 636–659.

Hsia, Y. E. (1977). Approaches to the appraisal of genetic counseling. *In* 'Genetic Counseling' (H. A. Lubs and F. de la Cruz, Eds), pp. 53–81. Raven Press, New York.

Janis, I. L. (1974). Vigilance and decision making in personal crises. *In* 'Coping and Adaptation' (D. A. Hamburg, C. V. Coelho and J. E. Adams, Eds), pp. 139–175. Basic Books, New York.

Janis, J. and Mann, L. (1977). 'Decision Making'. Free Press, New York.

Kallmann, F. J. (1956). Psychiatric aspects of genetic counseling. *Am. J. Hum. Genet.* **8**, 97–101.

Kassirer, J. P. and Pauker, S. G. (1981). The toss up. *N.E.J. Med.* **305**, 1467–1469.

Kessler, S. (1979). The genetic counselor as psychotherapist. *Birth Defects* **15**, 187–200.

Lippman-Hand, A. and Fraser, F. C. (1979). Genetic counseling – the postcounseling period: I. Parents' perceptions of uncertainty. *Am. J. Med. Genet.* **4**, 51–71.

Oakely, G. P., Jr., Brantley, K., Chan, A. T. L., Fernhoff, P. M., Goldberg, M. F., Priest, J. H. and Trusler, S. (1979). A community approach to prenatal diagnosis. *In* 'Services and Education in Medical Genetics' (F. H. Porter and E. B. Hook, Eds), pp. 163–182. Academic Press, New York.

Oetting, L. A. and Steele, M. W. (1982). A controlled retrospective follow up study of the impact of genetic counseling on parental reproduction following the birth of a Down syndrome child. *Clin. Genet.* **21**, 7–13.

Pauker, S. P. and Pauker, S. G. (1977). Prenatal diagnosis: a directive approach to genetic counseling using decision analysis. *Yale J. Biol. and Med.* **50**, 275–289.

Pearlin, L. I. and Schooler, C. (1978). The structure of coping. *J. Health and Soc. Behavior* **19**, 2–21.

Ransohoff, D. F. and Feinstein, A. R. (1976). Editorial: Is decision analysis useful in clinical medicine? *Yale J. Biol. and Med.* **49**, 165–168.

Sorenson, J. R., Sivazey, J. P. and Scotch, H. A. (1980). Birth Defects Conference on Fetus and the Newborn, New York.

Twiss, S. B. (1979). Problems of social justice in applied human genetics. *In* 'Genetic Counseling: Facts, Values and Norms' (A. M. Capron, R. F. Lappe, T. M. Murray, T. M. Powledge and D. Bergsma, Eds), pp. 255–277. A. R. Liss, New York.

Tversky, A. and Kahneman, D. (1974). Judgement under uncertainty: heuristics and biases. *Science* **185**, 1124–1131.

Tversky, A. and Kahneman, D. (1981). The framing of decisions and the psychology of choice, *Science* **211**, 453–458.

Weinstein, M. C. and Fineberg, H. V. (1980). 'Clinical Decision Analysis'. W. B. Saunders, Philadelphia.

4 Marital Pathology

JACK DOMINIAN

Introduction

The concept of marital pathology is a recent one. A number of observations have been made which have associated married partners with psychiatric disturbances. Thus in-patient, out-patient and general practice populations have all shown a higher-than-chance incidence of psychiatric disturbance in the spouse of patients. Other studies have shown a high incidence of parasuicide and suicide, alcoholism and violence associated with marital conflict. In general practice neurosis is associated with marital and family problems. All these clinical phenomena have been present in psychiatric literature for some forty years but no clear underlying pattern of pathology has emerged.

There has been theoretical speculation regarding the reasons for the presence of these clinical features. Extensive studies carried out in the United States in the forties and fifties have shown that as far as age at marriage, religious affiliation, social class, race and ethnic background are concerned, the process of selection is homogamy; that is to say like chooses like. This tendency for men and women to choose in each other characteristics similar to their own has been defined as assortative mating. One easy solution to the high incidence of psychiatric symptomatology in the spouses of psychiatric patients could be based on the theory of assortative mating. This would imply that one disturbed or potentially disturbed person chooses someone similar to themselves and thus both members are vulnerable to psychiatric disturbance from the very onset of the marriage. This would apply in particular to personality disorder or neurosis. In fact both American and British workers have advanced this proposition. Kreitman (1970) has challenged this view and shown that the degree of neurosis, as measured by an inventory, is the same as that of controls in spouses with high neurotic scores. In other words, established neurotics do not attract at the beginning of their marriage partners with an equal degree of neurosis. What Kreitman found is that the partners of neurotic spouses become as neurotic with the passage of time. His interpretation of this finding is that the process is not that of assortative mating but an interactional model. The neurotic spouse exercises an adverse effect on their normal partner. In a subsequent paper he showed that the sick spouse expects much greater face-to-face contact with their partner, restricting their association with the outside world and presumably raising their level of anxiety.

An alternative theory is that of Winch (1958) who proposed the principle of complementary needs. On this theory couples select one another on the basis of assortative mating for social factors but choose psychological characteristics of an opposite nature to their own as far as dominance, nurturing and achievement are concerned. This theory has been tested extensively and so far has not been confirmed.

Secondly there is the psychodynamic position. Basically this theory takes the view that there are two intimate relationships in life. The first is between ourselves and our parents and the second between ourselves and our spouse. The experiences of the first relationship influence that of the second. Basic patterns of deprivation, hostility, rejection, lack of self-esteem established in the first relationship are re-activated in the second, leading to conflict.

Finally there is the concept of a developmental cycle. Couples who marry in their late teens or early twenties have yet to clarify fully their identity. They marry with needs and expectations which will change with time and the stability of the relationship depends on the flexibility of the couple to accommodate each other as they proceed through the various phases of the life cycle.

In a series of papers I (Dominian, 1980) have tried to link these various theoretical models in one basic underlying concept, namely that the psychological pathology which emanates from marriage is the result of disturbance in the establishment and maintenance of the relationship which we call marriage. Marriage, or an equivalent intimate, permanent and exclusive relationship, is seen in terms of Bowlby's theory of human attachment with the formation and dissolution of the bond as the underlying theoretical model for marital pathology. Bowlby (1979) postulates that affect is involved in the formation of an intimate bond, another word for which would be love and that anxiety, depression and anger are experienced when an attachment is threatened or breaks down. The mobilization of these affective disturbances are at the root of the vast majority of psychiatric disturbance seen in practice.

Psychiatric disturbance in marital pathology

Before we look at affective disturbance during marriage itself, it is pertinent to refer to a study by Davies (1956) who some 30 years ago described 'engagement neurosis'. This is a condition characterized by manifestations of anxiety and depression and marked hesitation about the pending marriage. Now, it is true that a high proportion of couples about to get married get last minute apprehension feelings. These feelings are equally distributed between the sexes. They can be considered as normal reactions and the principal feature of such feelings is worry but no doubt or hesitation about the wedding.

In the escalated version of engagement neurosis the man or woman becomes so anxious or depressed that they cannot proceed with the wedding which is postponed. As soon as the postponement has taken place, the symptoms abate and the relationship is resumed with the same intensity until another date is fixed, when the symptoms return. The study referred to showed that, after five years, half of these patients were married but a quarter of the original group – whether married or not – continued to have fluctuating ill health.

Another unrecorded clinical observation which I think is related to engagement neurosis is the anxiety depression which may supervene swiftly to a spouse following a wedding ceremony in which the couple have either lived together before or not. The wedding ceremony imposes a stress, often the feeling that one cannot escape now, which is sufficient to trigger off an affective disorder of panic proportion. In some instances there is no recovery unless the relationship breaks up.

Whilst the early years of marriage are turbulent and may trigger off affective symptoms, there is one specific period which is crucial to the future of the relationship, namely the post puerperal phase. Most women experience transient maternal blues, a clinical feature of a passing depression. But in the overwhelming majority of cases, the symptoms clear up. In a few women, however, the symptoms persist and may combine with more severe manifestations of depression which arise in the first year after the birth of the baby (Pitt, 1973). The post-puerperal syndrome is characterized by loss of libido, lethargy, hostility and irritability to the spouse and a lowering of mood. Such a woman finds it very difficult to relate to her spouse sexually, emotionally or to cope with her household duties. If the syndrome persists, it tends to be highly damaging to the relationship. Nowadays antidepressants can change the picture swiftly, especially if coupled with an understanding attitude by the husband.

In the middle years of marriage, marital conflict takes the form in which one spouse – often the wife – is markedly unhappy in her marriage. She may wish to remain in it but radically alter her husband. She may wish to depart but finds it very difficult to face life alone. She may wish to go but does not want to break up the marriage for the sake of the children. In all these situations a progressive stress situation is set up which triggers off affective symptoms of anxiety and depression which may present either as psychological manifestations or psychosomatic features. When the situation continues to deteriorate, there may be violence, alcohol abuse and finally parasuicide. Many studies have shown that marital conflict is a prominent background factor for parasuicide (Bancroft 1977).

In the late years, that is some twenty or thirty years after the beginning of the marriage – when the children have grown up – one partner, usually the husband, may depart leaving behind a wife who is unable to cope with the loss of her spouse. Such women may enter into a prolonged depression which is incapable of being relieved, as they cannot accept or adapt to the loss of their partner.

Finally – and the most common pattern – is the depressive reaction to a departing spouse, at whatever stage of the marriage. In a retrospective study of 150 women who petitioned for divorce and had left their spouses, no fewer than 130 complained of symptoms suggestive of depression and the remaining twenty mentioned symptoms but did not consider them a disturbance of health (Chester, 1971). The one hundred and thirty women who complained of symptoms, mentioned in order of frequency, crying, weight change, sleep disturbance, tiredness, lack of concentration, increased smoking, self-neglect and drinking, all of which suggest a mixture of depression, anxiety and stress.

It is clear from this section that the major contribution to marital pathology comes from marital breakdown and so the features and size of this problem need to be described next.

Marital breakdown

Ever since divorce became a secular matter in the middle of the nineteenth century, there has been a steady rise in its incidence. This rise is not confined to the United Kingdom. A study of marital problems in Finland, Sweden, Norway, the Netherlands, Belgium, France, the Federal Republic of Germany, Switzerland, Austria and Italy all showed that divorce was increasingly common in every country and suggested that the causes were the same everywhere. Most of the countries showed a rise in incidence after the second world war, a decline in the fifties and then a constant upward trend after 1960 (Chester, 1977). Similar trends have been observed in the United States (Cherlin, 1981).

In England and Wales the number of decrees made absolute were 23 000 in 1960 and nearly 150 000 in 1980. The increase has been massive and when spouses and children are taken into consideration, some 500 000 men, women and children leave the courts annually. This constitutes a major social upheaval which contributes heavily to the ill-health of the community, both in terms of adult and child pathology.

Given the size of the problem, what do we know about the reasons which contribute to marital breakdown?

The reasons can be broadly divided into three. First there are major social changes affecting both sexes. The main change concerns women. There has been a persistent drive to raise the social status of women and one major result is that wives are no longer prepared to stay in marriages which appear to be intolerable or destructive to their personality. Continuing with the changes affecting women, since the end of the second world war there has been an upsurge of entry of women into the labour force, giving them a relative economic independence so that, if they wish to leave home, they are not entirely dependent on their husband. This independence has been reinforced by the smaller size family of an average two children which has been substantially contributed to by the advent of large-scale effective contraception. The rise of material standards in terms of food, shelter and – until recently – employment, has meant that expectations have also risen in the personal aspect of life with increased desire for emotional and sexual fulfilment. This increase of personal expectations in marriage has coincided with a reduction of religious affiliation and so the combination of this rise with a reduction of moral censure has aided divorce.

These are the broad social reasons and it can be seen that female emancipation is playing a major role. Within the context of these major changes in which couples expect so much more from marriage, certain specific social factors have been shown to be associated with divorce. Age has been shown to be an important factor. Teenage marriages are highly vulnerable and premarital pregnancy, particularly where it forced a marriage, is also associated with divorce. Social class and education show an inverse proportion, the lower the socio-economic grouping the higher the incidence of marital breakdown. All these factors have been studied in the United States and recently in Britain (Thornes and Collard, 1979). In this study social classes V and III (non-manual) are shown to be vulnerable. Marriages in which both partners are affiliated to a particular religion – and especially churchgoers – have a high degree of marital stability (Chester, 1977). Housing is also important. Disadvantaged housing, especially in the early years of marriage, is associated with divorce (Thornes and Collard, 1979). Childless couples are more prone to divorce and early fertility is associated with serious marital difficulty (Thornes and Collard, 1979).

Finally, the third group of reasons are related to interpersonal conflict in which there is a failure to fulfil the minimal affectionate and sexual needs of one or both partners. Whilst social reasons predispose to marital vulnerability, couples survive these handicaps provided their personal relationship fulfils their minimum needs. Thus, when one finally meets the couple who are seriously upset with one another, the presenting features will indicate that the ultimate cause for their frustration and disappointment is emotional and sexual. The patterns of these disturbances will be considered later in this review.

One feature stands out in the findings of research. This is the timing of marital breakdown. The marital problems of those who divorce start early. By the second anniversary 52 per cent of the marital problems had appeared and by the fifth anniversary, 73 per cent. These figures appertain to all divorced persons. There is, however, a marked difference between the sexes. By the first anniversary women recognize some 44 per cent of problems as against only 23 per cent by men. By the fifth anniversary, women have recognized 80 per cent of the marital problems whilst men only 60 per cent. Thus marital problems appear early, are recognized much earlier by women and there is overwhelming evidence that it is wives who want to intervene and remedy as opposed to their husbands who want to procrastinate (Brannen and Collard, 1982). In fact nearly half of all divorces occur in the first nine years of marriage and, since the actual separation took place some three years before, the vulnerability of the first six years of marriage is most marked. Research has shown that whenever divorce occurs in the first twenty years of marriage, the start of the major problems occurred for half of the couples in the first five years of marriage. All this has important implications for marriage which needs particular protection and support in its early years.

Patterns of marital pathology

There is no agreed coherent picture of marital pathology. As already stated there are several theories which have not been combined into a comprehensive whole. What follows is a pattern of marital pathology, constructed by myself (Dominian, 1980) and based on the life cycle of family life. The idea is that marriage goes through several phases and the needs of the couple change with time. The present presentation is based on a combination of various dimensions of behaviour in various phases of marriage. The phases of marriage are shortened into three. Phase I covers the first five years of marriage which normally end at about the age of thirty. The second phase covers the next twenty years of marriage ending at fifty and coinciding with the growth of children and the menopause of the wife; and the third phase spans the period between fifty and the death of one partner. Each phase is considered under five parameters affecting the social, physical, emotional, intellectual and spiritual aspect of the relationship. The events which occur in each phase predominate during it but are no means exclusive. There is a good deal of overlap, but the schema allows a clarification of what is happening.

Phase I

Social aspects

The social factors involve the withdrawal from parents and friends, the setting up of a home, constructing a life within it, arranging the chores and finding a satisfactory financial, work and leisure arrangement. Conflict can arise in all these areas.

At the very heart of the marital relationship is the establishment of an intimate relationship between husband and wife. In order to achieve this the couple have to maintain friendly relations with their parents but not allow them to dictate or interfere with their newly established rapport. In-laws – particularly mothers-in law – provide problems early in marriage (Blood and Wolfe, 1960). They do this by intruding into the decision making of the spouses and taking sides with their offspring against their partner, particularly when they feel hostile towards them (Thornes and Collard, 1979). The same applies to friends. Couples will retain some friends with whom they had established close contact before marriage and they will drop others. A particularly retained friend may have special meaning, being an ex- boy or girl friend and may be a source of jealousy. Such a person may have to be given up but care should be taken to ensure that this jealousy is not a manifestation of a deeper desire to isolate and exclude the spouse from his/her friends.

Couples who acquire their own households have to establish its running. Nowadays men are expected to do much more in the house and many do. Some promise a great deal before marriage and then do very little afterwards. In practice wives are prepared to take the major share of household duties but they feel particularly upset if their spouse promises a lot and then lets them down. A special form of complaint is to be found in those couples where the husband undertakes to redecorate, do up a bathroom or kitchen and takes an extraordinary long time to do it whilst he is ready to help the neighbourhood immediately.

Money is a frequently mentioned problem at any time of the marriage but the seeds of disillusion are sown in these early years. The wife is the spouse who complains most frequently that her husband is mean or keeps her short of money. In addition to its economic significance money has also an emotional value. The wife often feels that if she was loved she would not be subjected to such deprivation.

At the beginning of marriage both spouses are working and this produces considerable fatigue in the wife who has also to take the bulk of the household caring responsibility. The husband's work may provide special problems.

These are often connected with working late, leaving little time to see his family, and talk to them. Not only may he work late, but a perennial complaint of the wife is that he does not inform her of his late arrival and all her cooking plans go astray. When he comes home he may bring work with him or, feeling tired, may have a meal and simply sit in front of the TV in a semi-mesmerized way, impervious to the presence of his wife or children. Another problem is connected with the man who has to spend a good deal of his time away.

Finally in these early years of marriage, the husband may not only work hard but use all his spare time to be with his friends at the pub, sportsfield or following his favourite hobby. This is the man who marries and wants to enjoy the privileges of marriage whilst maintaining the freedom of the bachelor life. The combination often proves intolerable to the wife who needs companionship.

Physical

The sexual side of marriage is assuming increasing importance in the minimum requirements of marriage. A couple expect to enjoy their sexual life even if it is not perfect in every respect. Workers in the United States have reported that 82 per cent of wives married for less than a year find their sexual life good or very good and this figure increases to 88 per cent when the wives could communicate fully with their spouse about their reactions and feelings (Levin and Levin, 1975). That still leaves 12 to 18 per cent dissatisfied, which agrees closely with a British study which found that 12 to 20 per cent of wives were initially sexually dissatisfied (Thornes and Collard, 1979). This dissatisfaction may be accounted for by poor preparation for love-making, inadequate technique, infrequent intercourse or, more specifically, sexual dysfunction including non-consummation, premature ejaculation and impotence. The wife may develop her own specific problems which are failure to achieve orgasm, inability to relax with dyspareunia and occasionally complete disgust with sex.

Sexual difficulties at the start of the marriage rarely precipitate marital disruption; couples hope that the situation will improve and often it does. Sexual satisfaction is however an important contributor to marital happiness (Gebhard, 1966) and, if the performance does not improve, becomes infrequent or ceases, then the relationship gradually suffers. In particular this applies to the persistent loss of libido and therefore infrequent intercourse in the process of protracted post-puerperal depression.

Extramarital intercourse is not common in these early years but it may occur in marriages in which the spouses had a very active sex life with each other and others prior to marriage or when one spouse – usually the husband

– has a job which takes him away from home frequently and sometimes – to the acute distress of the wife – when she is pregnant and cannot have intercourse. In his study Eysenck (1978) has suggested that the stable extrovert with high libido and the unstable introvert with low libido with strong inhibitions are both likely to have extramarital activity.

The outcome of adultery depends entirely on the response of the spouse. At this early stage of the marriage, forgiveness is common but at the same time mistrust can set in.

The advent of children introduces a major change in the marital relationship. The couple now change from being a dyad to a triad and the presence of a child introduces a new dimension of joy in marriage. But all is not joy. The mother experiences far more fatigue (Wiegand and Gross, 1958) and this may alter her total availability to her husband who now complains that his wife is totally immersed in her children and has no time for him or for socialising.

Emotional

In addition to sexual fulfilment, the exchange of adequate affection is the other key element in a satisfactory marital relationship. This exchange depends on adequate communication and effective expression of loving feelings. The lack of affection is one of the commonest complaints in marital problems. Wives complain that husbands do not talk to them or do not show their loving feelings even when they truly love them. In particular, wives state that husbands who do not express loving feelings expect sexual intercourse and this depersonalized approach makes them feel they are treated as sexual objects.

Next to communication of affection comes the resolution of conflict. All marriages will experience conflict and its resolution is an essential component of marital stability. Unresolved conflict leads to verbal aggression and ultimately to physical aggression (Gayford, 1975). Short of verbal and physical aggression is the presence of acute sensitivity in one or both spouses. The sensitive spouse hates criticism, cannot accept responsibility for anything done wrong and, when accused, often withdraws into a long sulk or angrily denies the accusation. When both couples behave like this, constant rows are the order of the day.

There are, however, some specific emotional problems which appear early in marriage and involve attachment, trust and dependence.

Bowlby (1979) has written extensively about factors in childhood which lead to anxious attachments. These are men and women who find it very difficult to establish and maintain sustained relationships. They are always on their guard that they will be rejected or let down and find it very difficult to believe that another person really wants them. These characteristics are also features of the affectless, psychopathic personality and such people may drop out of a marital relationship very early on.

The principal feature of these men and women is a low degree of trust. They expect to be let down and hurt. If their spouse commits adultery or lets them down in one of the patterns of social behaviour already described, their initial low trust drops further and they may refuse to continue in the relationship.

The other factor is emotional dependence. This element plays a crucial part in marital disharmony. Men and women should reach marriage having emancipated themselves from their emotional link with their parents. They should be, up to a point, self-reliant, self-directing, self-governing, able to take responsibility for their lives, cope with adversity and be able both to receive and express affection. There are marriages when neither partner has reached this stage of development and both are trying to make the other a parental figure, a role neither can play and such marriages are not viable.

Sometimes both husband and wife are rebelling against their parents and their only common bond is their mutual rejection of parents, which is not a sufficient basis for the maintenance of the relationship. But the commonest pattern is one in which one partner is the dependent one. If it is the husband his wife will complain that he refuses to take decisions and thrusts all of them on to her. He is passive and refuses to take the initiative. He avoids responsibility in dealing with letters, bills and is financially inept. He simply expects his wife to carry on where his parents left off. Very often such a man marries a woman who appears strong and reliant and is dominant in the belief that her strength will sustain him. There are, however, complications in this choice. Often he is not only dependent on his wife but resentful and aggressive towards her authority, which he needs and resents at the same time. The other problem is that often the apparently 'strong' woman has behavioural characteristics of strength such as a commanding voice, an assertive manner, a brusque approach and yet is herself anxious and insecure underneath, what Eysenck would call an anxious extrovert, and so her appearance belies her true weakness.

Similarly it may be the wife who is emotionally dependent. This is much more common and much more acceptable in our culture, but it has its problems later on as we shall see in the second phase. In the meantime severe emotional dependence on the husband is resented at an early stage. Such a wife finds it difficult to cook, shop, look after the house or after the children and relies on her husband to do all these things. She is in constant contact with her family, visits them frequently and continues to use them as her principal advisers.

Such emotional dependence may be associated with a high degree of anxiety leading to two other recurrent features present in marital pathology;

namely jealousy and possessiveness. The anxious dependent husband or wife is living constantly with the fear of being abandoned. They are extremely suspicious of others and express this in the form of jealousy. Jealousy is not entirely contributed to by dependence and the fear of abandonment; the sufferer has often also low self-esteem. The combination of low self-esteem, dependence and the fear of abandonment makes such men not only jealous but also possessive. They try to isolate their partner from their family, friends and acquaintances and keep them entirely to themselves. If possible they would have their partner under lock and key all the time. Such jealous spouses complain bitterly that their partner was flirting at parties, has imaginary affairs and, if it is the wife, she is accused of behaving like a 'whore' when she even looks at another man.

These problems are frequently found in marital discord and show the intimate link between marital pathology and personality disorder.

Intellectual

Usually an adequate courtship will ensure that a couple share a common background and mutual interests, so that intellectually they are matched in their daily concerns. If there has been no adequate courtship or the marriage has been enacted in a hurry, then a couple may soon find that they have nothing in common and they become bored with each other.

Spiritual

Studies in the forties and fifties suggested that mixed religious marriages were vulnerable to marital breakdown. This phenomenon has probably become less now as more and more marriages are mixed, particularly between Christian denominations. Nevertheless, a common spiritual background in terms of churchgoing or common shared values strengthens the bond. When couples vary markedly in their values regarding fidelity, permanency, honesty, and integrity, then respect wanes and the partner loses gradually his/her significance.

Phase II

The second phase, which covers approximately the years between 30 and 50 and also on average overlaps the fifth and twenty-fifth years of marriage, is most important because during this period some 60 per cent of divorces occur (Social Trends, 1976). During this phase the problems referred to in the first phase may continue and become unacceptable or new ones emerge. The particular feature of the new problems is associated with change either in social circumstances or in the personality.

Social

During this phase most couples have established permanent abodes with a certain measure of stability. People working in the armed forces, foreign civil service and some business personnel may change homes at regular intervals and this may contribute to instability.

A particular problem of these years is upward or downward mobility. It is the husband who is usually successful and may climb into a different social network. In this network the wife may or may not fit and, if she does not, she is left behind. This is painful to her but it is particularly distasteful when she sacrificed her money, time or even career at the start of the marriage to promote her husband's interest. Downward social mobility may follow persistent unemployment, drinking, gambling or imprisonment. All these adverse social factors are associated with high divorce rates. The recent high rate of unemployment has yet to show itself in marital breakdown figures.

Physical

An already quoted British study has shown that in a sample of continued married men and women, 98 per cent of the former and 96 per cent of the latter claimed that the sexual side of their marriage either started and continued satisfactorily or earlier difficulties had been resolved. Whereas in 38 per cent of divorced women and 30 per cent of divorced men whose initial sexual relationship was said to be good, this deteriorated with the passage of time (Thornes and Collard, 1979). Most of this deterioration occurs during these years. Partners who subsequently divorce tend to blame the other partner for being 'selfish' or 'inconsiderate' (complaints mostly by women), 'cold' (complaint mostly by men) and 'cruel' (mentioned entirely by women). Selfishness and cruelty include: reaching a climax quickly without concern for the wife, making love when drunk, forcing intercourse against the wish of the wife, persistent demands for an unacceptable sexual variation and too frequent demands by the husband.

The majority of extramarital sex occurs during these years and if a spouse has more than one affair the partner may find such conduct unacceptable.

Emotional

Perhaps the single most important pattern of emotional upheaval follows the emotional maturation of the dependent partner. Since it is the wife who is most commonly involved in this growth, her typical story is described. Such a wife finds that in the first phase of marriage she is willing to be compliant to her husband's wishes. Then gradually and imperceptibly she begins to rebel. Now she wants to take her life in her hands. She wants to drive the car, have her own circle of friends, decide where they are going for their holidays, wants to know how much her husband is earning and desires to have a say how the money is spent. She may desire to go to work against her husband's wishes, insist on much less criticism towards her and a good deal of serious consideration of her wishes.

At the same time she becomes much more critical of her husband, resents his dominance and bossiness and answers back. In brief she now wants to be acknowledged as an adult partner and not as a child. Most husbands adapt to this common change. There are, however, a few who do not. They refuse to accept the change and are genuinely puzzled by the emerging personality of their wife. Their refusal to accept the change leads to arguments and quarrels. The wife angrily withdraws affection and sex until the husband yields. If he does not, she turns elsewhere for recognition of her newly found status and she describes how she falls out of love with her husband and in love with somebody else. Or she may simply leave the matrimonial home because she has had enough of being dominated. Often when she does that the husband suddenly capitulates and is prepared to concede everything. By now it is too late and this pattern of marital breakdown contributes largely to divorce during these years.

Intellectual and spiritual

Unilateral change may also occur in both these fields. Spouses may develop different interests and priorities so that they come to have little in common.

Phase III

The third phase of marriage extends from about the age of fifty to the death of one spouse, a period that may span twenty years or more and is a phenomenon of increasing frequency in this century.

Social

The main social event of this period is the departure of children, their marriage and the change of parents into grandparents. The departure of children allows the couple more time to themselves and studies have shown a return to the original level of satisfaction in the marriage in this phase. It is a phase often accompanied with material well-being and freedom from anxiety coupled finally with retirement of the spouses, allowing an even greater intimacy. The main contribution to marital breakdown is the departure of children. Couples with low personal satisfaction in marriage have stayed together until their children have grown up and then find no further reason for doing so.

Physical

Recent work has shown that sexual activity continues in the sixties and seventies and expectations for this continuity are part of contemporary marriage. Women, now freed from the anxieties of pregnancy, have a renewed interest in sexual intercourse whose frequency abates but whose loving and meaning is enhanced. The menopause has no effect on the frequency or enjoyment of sexual intercourse but wives with existing premenopausal sexual problems may use the menopause as an excuse for dissatisfaction with their marriage and giving up sex (Ballinger, 1976). Another problem affects the male. Kinsey (1948) was the first worker to show increased impotence with age and such impotence may be a disturbing factor in the marriage, giving the wife anxiety feelings that she is no longer loved or that her husband is having an affair. In these circumstances the husband should compensate for his impotence by giving his wife greater affection.

Emotional

Three patterns of marital emotional difficulties are seen in this phase. The first consists of problems which have existed since the beginning of the marriage. The second are the continuing ones from Phase II in which one partner is asserting independence and has reached a point of wishing to depart. The third is linked with the departure of children. The couple are now left with no interest to hide their emotional emptiness which is recognized for the first time. The departure of children is a signal for the dissolution of some marriages that were only held together by their presence.

Intellectual and spiritual

In this phase – as in the second – couples may go their separate ways developing different outlooks and values. This independence may split the marriage when there is no underlying emotional or sexual unity.

Counselling

General principles

Counselling in marital problems was initially a process by which the spouses were seen individually by different counsellors. Increasingly it has been recognized that it is the couple together who need help and nowadays the emphasis is placed on one or two counsellors seeing the couple together. The commonest pattern of therapy is for one counsellor alone to see a couple. By doing this he can watch the interaction of husband and wife. Feelings of anger, hostility, anxiety, periods of silence, manner of communication are all noted and commented upon as indicated. The usual problem of listening to a one-sided interpretation is corrected by the presence of both partners who interject and give their own version of what happened. In this way the counsellor can see that the spouse who complains of being a victim of their partner's indifference, neglect, hostility may in fact unconsciously provoke this behaviour and so a better understanding of the interaction takes place.

When a couple are seen for the first time, note is taken of which spouse starts talking first and generally the pattern of communication. Gradually the story of the marriage unfolds and the respective contributions to the problems are appraised. Often spouses come to such a session to pour out all their complaints and get the counsellor on their side. Counselling is clearly not a question of taking sides, judging or criticizing. The role of the counsellor is to show the couple their mutual needs and the way they are failing to meet these requirements. The role of emotions is vital and much marital conflict is due to excessive destructive criticism and not enough praise, affirmation or affection. The counsellor will help the couple see this and help them retrace their steps to achieve it. In doing this the counsellor will inject a ray of hope and encouragement in an otherwise embittered and disillusioned relationship. Couples will be seen on enough occasions to bring about sufficient change so that they are set on a new course. In order for this to take place the counsellor needs to be conversant with the principles of marital pathology so that, by the end of the first session, he can show the couple that he really understands their predicament by spelling out accurately the emotionally disturbed pattern of interaction. Sometimes this type of insight therapy is not possible and the couple have to be given more explicit instructions on how to communicate and reward each other in a behaviouristic model of therapy (Stuart, 1969). In this type of therapy the basic principle is, 'If you do this for me, I will do this for you'. Behaviour is changed without insight.

One spouse

The ideal is to work with a couple who are motivated to change. In practice two problems arise. Firstly both partners will not always come and secondly, when they do come, one or both are not interested in change. They have already made up their minds that no change is possible and expecting nothing from the interview they have already made alternative plans, including the decision to go. Thus the initial motivation to change and stay in the marriage is crucial for the outcome.

Often only one spouse will seek help. This is frequently the wife whose husband will not come. With her permission such a husband can be written to in non-threatening terms and invited to come. Sometimes this works. When it does not, one is left to work with one spouse who is often the wife. In these circumstances such a patient can be listened to and much accomplished with her. Thus, if her husband has accused her of being 'mad' she can be reassured about her sanity. If she lacks confidence to stand up to her husband, she can be given this. If she wants to leave and needs support to achieve this, she can be supported to achieve it. Sometimes her improvement challenges her husband who comes along out of envy or curiosity. Most often the wife is helped to understand herself and her husband so that she can facilitate his life. Thus, whilst the ideal is to see and help the couple, something can be accomplished with the single spouse.

Conclusions

The essence of marriage counselling is the ability to help a couple see and understand the distortion of their marital encounter. The counsellor remains emotionally detached but friendly and concerned and, without taking sides, facilitates the spouses to gain insight of their particular interaction on the basis of his social and dynamic knowledge of intimate human relationships.

References

Ballinger, C. B. (1976). 'Psychiatric morbidity and the menopause: clinical features'. *Br. Med. J.* **1**, 1183–1185.

Bancroft, J., Skrimshire, A., Casson, J., Harvard-Watt, O., Reynolds, F. (1977). People who deliberately poison or injure themselves: their problems and their contacts with helping agencies. *Psychol. Med.* **7**, 289–303.

Blood, R. O. and Wolfe, D. M. (1960). 'Husbands and Wives: The Dynamics of Married Living'. Free Press, New York.

Bowlby, J. (1979). 'The Making and Breaking of Affectional Bonds'. Tavistock Publications, London.

Brannen, J. and Collard, J. (1982). 'Marriages in Trouble'. Tavistock Publications, London.

Cherlin, A. J. (1981). 'Marriage, Divorce, Remarriage'. Harvard University Press, London.

Chester, R. (1971). 'Health and Marriage Breakdown: Experience of a Sample of Divorced Women'. *Br. J. Preventive Soc. Med.* **25**, 231–235.

Chester, R. (Editor) (1977). 'Divorce in Europe'. Martinus Nijhoff Social Services Division, London.

Davies, D. L. (1956). 'Psychiatric Illness in the Engaged to be Married'. *Br. J. Preventive Soc. Med.* **10**, 123–127.

Dominian, J. (1980). 'Marital Pathology'. Darton Longman and Todd/British Medical Association, London.

Eysenck, H. J. (1978). 'Sex and Personality'. Abacus, London.

Gayford, J. J. (1975). 'Wife Battering: a Preliminary Survey of 100 Cases'. *Br. Med. J.* **1**, 194–197.

Gebhard, P. H. (1966). 'Factors in Marital Orgasm'. *J. Soc. Issues* **22**, 88–95.

Kinsey, A. C. (1948). 'Sexual Behaviour in the Human Male'. Saunders and Co., London.

Kreitman, N. (1970). 'Neurosis and Marital Interaction'. *Br. J. Psychiatry* **117**, 33–46.

Levin, R. J. and Levin, A. (1975). 'Sexual Pleasure, the Surprising Preferences of 10 000 Women'. Redbook, New York.

Pitt, B. (1973). 'Maternity Blues'. *Br. J. Psychiatry* **122**, 431–433.

Social Trends (1976). HMSO, London.

Stuart, R. B. (1969). 'Interpersonal treatment for marital discord'. *J. Consult. Clin. Psychol.* **33**, 675–682.

Thornes, B. and Collard, J. (1979). 'Who Divorces?'. Routledge, Keegan and Paul, London.

Wiegand, E. and Gross, I. H. (1958). 'Fatigue of Homemakers with Young Children'. *Tech. Bull.* 265. Michigan Agricultural Experiment Station.

Winch, R. F. (1958). 'Male Selection: A Study of Complementarity Needs.' Harper, New York.

5 Early Infant Loss and Multiple Congenital Abnormalities

KERRY BLUGLASS

Introduction – the counselling task

Bereavement counselling has both similarities to and differences from genetic counselling. Physicians, paediatricians and geneticists who are skilled in providing detailed and informative genetic counselling will be practised at providing information, the first requisite of effective counselling. But giving the parents or the family didactic and directive information and instruction are not of themselves sufficient. The 'counselling' approach must include more than this, and different skills have to be acquired.

Some of these skills involved in counselling are now being taught much more frequently to medical students at an early stage of their career, and so are more available to newly qualified doctors. Also training is commonly available on counselling courses (for example, those run by the College of General Practitioners, Regional Postgraduate Centres, and so on). For less recently qualified doctors this may seem to involve a new and unfamiliar way of dealing with the family or parents, a way that at first sight seems more time consuming, but which in the long run can be shown to be much more effective.

This approach involves more listening and less talking (making allowances for the fact that solid information nevertheless has to be conveyed as explained above). It involves allowing the patient or the family time to reflect on matters under discussion, and much more use of open ended questions than has been traditional in a medical consultation.

Example: Closed question (traditional medical consultation), 'Have you been quite well recently?'

Example: Open ended question, 'Tell me what you feel about your recent health?'

It can be seen that the first example usually elicits the answer 'Yes' or 'No', while the second example requires the patient or parent to formulate some thoughts on the subject and allows them to reflect on their feelings.

The counsellor has to try to recall continually that every patient or parent is an individual, with a unique previous life experience as well as individual personality make-up, intellectual level and experience, and that the aim should be for the counsellor to help the parent to arrive at an informed state where he or she can make plans and decisions, rather than have the counsellor impose them upon the patient or make some for him or her. This may sound self evident and simplistic, but this is quite a different style of consultation to the more familiar organic, medical, consultation in which a diagnosis is reached, instructions are given in a directive fashion about treatment, and factual information is conveyed about prognosis and outcome. Of course, the task of the genetic counsellor must include the giving of factual information about disease processes, statistical likelihood of recurrence and treatment and prognosis for say, an affected child, but where a child has been lost or where the 'perfect' expected child has been born with a handicap, the directive approach has to be modified to suit the situation as far as the bereavement is concerned. This adaptation of approach will enable the counsellor better to appreciate the impact of the loss on the parents' decisions and plans for the future.

Early infant loss

The range of clinical situations which the genetic counsellor will encounter in clinical practice range from the death of a child in early infancy from such disorders as neural tube defect and other congenital malformations, through death in the perinatal and post-perinatal periods, to the earliest reproductive losses, as for example in intra-uterine death and even the loss of an early pregnancy by spontaneous or therapeutic abortion.

In some instances of course, the couple or parent requiring advice or counselling may have experienced more than one of these events, or a recurrence of a particular one.

Until recently, particularly with the growth in interest in maternal–infant bonding or attachment, it had generally been assumed that the longer the period of gestation or the older the baby or live infant, the more closely and realistically the mother would have bonded to the baby and therefore the greater the feelings of bereavement if a baby did not survive. However, it is now known that not all births of live, healthy babies result in immediate, ideal attachment, a bond which is only disrupted by death. Even if this were the case, the knowledge that a baby may not survive or has a progressive disease which is likely to prove fatal within weeks or months, or has a severe congenital malformation, may be accompanied by a process of adaptation to the impending loss, or 'anticipatory grieving'. This, as will be discussed in this chapter, brings both benefits and disadvantages, but for the moment it can be assumed to mitigate some aspects of the loss.

Conversely, the parent who is pregnant and loses the baby early on, for example a first or second trimester loss, should not necessarily be assumed to have a less severe reaction to bereavement in proportion with the period of gestation.

Far more important is the significance of the pregnancy to the mother or parents, her or their previous experience of loss and adaptation to it, previous personality and social support.

Example: The wife of a doctor experienced much unexpected anguish and distress following a spontaneous miscarriage so early in pregnancy that foetal movements had not yet been felt. She and her husband were quite unprepared for the sense of loss and disappointment, 'social failure' and even hostile comment from acquaintances – 'You must have done something . . .'. This was heightened by many work-mates who were pregnant at the time. She was a stable young woman however and adapted quickly to the situation.

Bereavement is now accepted as a 'Life Event' to which the majority of people adapt in an individual way, given time and adequate support, but which may in vulnerable individuals precipitate morbidity (in physical as well as psychological terms), or even mortality in some. There is now evidence that effective counselling for the bereaved prevents some of the worst morbidity and mitigates other aspects, so that psychosocial outcome can be considerably improved.

The need for support and counselling should be seen in the context of the twentieth century where customary and traditional support previously derived from formal religious beliefs as well as close and supportive family networks and more social acceptance of death and funerals, are now lacking. Professionals are concerned, not to turn grieving and loss into illness, which indeed it is not, being a 'normal' process, if now less commonly encountered, but rather in our present approach to preventive medicine, to look for ways in which to prevent psychosocial morbidity and illness in the vulnerable, or potentially vulnerable, members of the population.

The timing of intervention is most important. Early identification of parents or families at risk or potentially in need of help will improve outcome. For this reason, parents should be assessed and kept in close touch with the counsellor or counselling team as soon as possible after the death of the baby, rather than allow a long interval to elapse before follow-up, during which difficulties may have developed and abnormal patterns entrenched, or pathological mourning established.

Following any loss, which may include death of a partner, loss of a parent, amputation of a limb or of a breast, certain psychological processes are usually experienced. As with descriptions of the psychological processes involved when a patient is aware that he or she is dying, it should not be assumed that these stages or processes will always follow in a certain order and that a repetition or regression to an earlier stage necessarily must mean abnormality (Table 5.1).

Table 5.1   Stages of bereavement

Shock, disbelief, numbness – often followed by profound physical discomfort; stomach pains, aching limbs, etc.
Pining and yearning
Depression of spirits and apathy
Bargaining and mitigation – the 'if only' stage
Anger, guilt

For a detailed review of bereavement and grieving, the reader should consult Parkes (1972).

However, until fairly recently, what was known of loss in general and bereavement in particular, chiefly derived from studies of widows and widowers. Certain features are indeed common to the loss of a partner and the loss of any other family member, for example, feelings of guilt, self-reproach, hostility, anger, depression and sadness. What is less clear, is the extent to which other factors may prolong or mitigate the adaptation. Whereas it is commonly held that the period of adaptation to loss after the death of a spouse may be complete in approximately one year to fifteen months or so, it may have a more protracted course. Clinical practice (Bluglass, 1982) suggests that some parents may continue to mourn a lost child for a very much longer period before resolution is complete, without necessarily being in a stage of pathological grief. However, it must be said that as clinicians we tend to see 'clinic' populations and not populations as a whole. Much less is known about families who do adapt and resolve the loss of a child, and indeed there is insufficient evidence about those families who will require intensive intervention and those who will manage very well without. For this reason, good practice suggests that the availability of intervention and attention to the potential needs of the parents merits consideration, since prevention is considerably better and more effective than cure.

The effect on the family

The parents

Regardless of the clinical causes, the death of a live infant, a stillbirth or the loss of a baby earlier in pregnancy may have severe repercussions on the parents. In turn, parents have to relate to and support and interact with each other and other family members.

The psychological process of adapting to loss, grieving, and mourning is a complex one and requires time, concentration and much physical and emotional energy. This is often forgotten. The physical and psychosomatic effects of grieving can be powerful, and their effect sapping of energy normally reserved for other tasks, for example, domestic, occupational, parenting and so on.

Thus a parent may actually accomplish the grieving process painfully but adequately, but have no resources left effectively to interact with, let alone be supportive to, his or her marital partner. In this way common and normal feelings of guilt, accusation (however irrational and unfounded) may be readily magnified or imputed to the other partner, with a deterioration in relationships. There is clinical evidence that alterations in general health, alcohol, tobacco and medication use, may further aggravate the situation.

Because of the understanding of the close bond between mother and baby it has often been assumed that mothers will suffer most, and usually attention is directed by relatives, friends and family physicians to the well-being of the mother. In contemporary society, especially in the UK, less expectation is made of the effects of grief on fathers, particularly for the loss of a very young infant or one in the neonatal period. Clinical experience with a large number of bereaved parents in one study (Bluglass, 1982) has demonstrated that where fathers do not openly grieve, or suppress their grief, a potentially hazardous form of consolation and solace is in increasing alcohol consumption, and it can be seen that this in itself is not only dangerous to health but can exacerbate fragile marital relations.

Traditionally, the man is expected to be strong and support the grieving mother. It may, therefore, be very difficult for a father, particularly if young and relatively inexperienced, to declare his own need for support and advice.

Example: Following the death of a baby, two fathers in one series became excessively preoccupied with their own health, one developing a fear of cancer and the other multiple hypochondriacal symptoms.

In the same study, a father whose baby had died at the age of one month did not openly express grief, but when seen a few months later his alcohol consumption was assuming dangerous proportions and he had twice crashed a car while under the influence of alcohol. He also complained of many physical symptoms, headaches and other ailments for which no cause other than severe tension was found.

In general, the normal process of grief and mourning is not necessarily synonymous with clinical depression, but on occasions it can certainly look very similar, and what is more important, it may have a similar impact on the surviving children. Withdrawal, apathy, poor concentration, insomnia and irritability may all be present singly or in combination at different stages of bereavement and will affect the functioning of a parent.

The children

The damaging impact of a 'sick' parent on the development and behaviour of children is well described in the literature (Rutter, 1966), especially where the parental illness involves withdrawal of interest, affection and care, as opposed to more frankly psychotic features.

It is thus very important to identify and treat depressive symptoms when present and to try to mitigate the effects of grieving on the children themselves. This may involve the intervention of another family member who is less affected. A friend, neighbour, teacher or other professional person may temporarily provide for the child or children of the family the warmth and interest which the grieving parent is unable to provide. The child or children in addition will be exposed to the feelings of loss of the baby either explicitly, or as implied by the parents. This can be bewildering for children who sense an altered atmosphere but where, for example, in the case of an early miscarriage or a death *in utero* nearer to term the reason for the parental sadness is not explained to them.

Where the baby has survived long enough to come home and join the family unit, a very young child may not fully understand the death and may, due to his developmental age, by a process of 'primitive' or 'magical' thinking, believe that he himself caused the disappearance of the baby, or may believe that the disease which killed the dead child will in turn kill him.

Other, often older children may simply experience the family feelings of loss, but if this cannot be fully expressed and shared, if the opportunity to ask questions and be comforted are not available, substantial emotional problems and reactions may develop. These may range in severity from transient fears and phobias to more serious neurotic and behaviour problems.

Example. A little girl experienced the loss of two baby brothers in infancy. Her mother complained that she frequently played with an imaginary baby in her bedroom, laying out toys, clothes, feeding utensils for it, and reassuring the fantasy baby that she, the surviving sibling, would take care of the baby better than her mother who had 'allowed' two previous babies to die. Not surprisingly, this behaviour was distressing and indeed alarming for the parents.

Mourning and expression of grief

Parents seeking advice often ask whether it is appropriate or wise to take children to funerals. Clearly where children are very small, for example, as in the toddler period, or where there is no actual funeral or ceremony as in the case of babies not deemed to have lived, i.e. stillbirths, this is more readily solved. However, psychiatrists and others working intensively with bereaved families now usually feel that the opportunity to attend a funeral and to experience a 'leave taking' is a part of learning about life and facilitates healthy grieving. If the child's first experience of a funeral and death can be one where the deceased is not a close family relative or when the death of such a relative is the first experienced by a child but a friend or less involved family member can be there to support the child, then it is usually helpful and not harmful. The support of a person outside the family or one less involved would be essential if, for example, the child's parent had died, since the surviving parent would clearly be much too involved in practical matters and his or her own grief to support the child or children adequately. A helpful relative or friend can fulfill this function.

What does seem to be important, however, is the acknowledgement of tears and sadness as being appropriate and not harmful at this stage. There has been for some time a belief that to allow tears to be shed by the recently bereaved, or indeed the less recently bereaved, was somehow damaging or harmful to the individual concerned. It has been this belief which has so often resulted in professionals encouraging the suppression of grief and society in general forbidding tears or other expressions of sadness with exhortations to 'cheer up', 'not to think so morbidly', and in the case of a lost baby, exhortations to 'never mind, dear, you're still young, you can have another one'.

Only listening to the feelings, thoughts and expressions of the needs of the bereaved sufficiently often will disclose that there is frequently a need to cry, to talk about the deceased and to find an accepting atmosphere where the bereaved person is not 'hushed up'. This is, of course, true for people in the early or intermediate stages of grief, although when we consider pathological responses to grieving it will be seen that chronic unresolved grieving is another matter.

When parents lose a baby, particularly if it is the first in the family, it is understandable that they themselves may wish to have another child as soon as possible (unless positively advised against it).

Their surrounding family members and friends may exhort them to do so believing that this is helpful advice. For many mothers who were looking forward to the birth of a baby and had a fruitless pregnancy, the strong biological urge to be pregnant again and to hope for a more successful outcome is very natural.

However, many people are nevertheless uncertain about their own feelings and it does seem that some parents try again for another pregnancy in the belief that a strong recommendation to this effect has been given by their obstetrician, paediatrician, or family doctor.

This recalls what was said earlier about counselling, since some attention to, and acceptance of, the expressed feelings of the parents at this stage may disclose that they are still very actively grieving for the infant they have lost. Over-dogmatic advice to have another child as soon as possible may present problems in various ways: it certainly seems that being in the active stages of mourning and grieving involving affective (mood) changes very like depression, may be physiologically undesirable in pregnancy. This may account for the reference in some studies to repeated miscarriage or failure to carry to term following an earlier infant loss. Although perhaps this association is difficult to prove, one would try in pregnancy to avoid situations in which the mothers were known to be subject to more anxiety, stress or increase in smoking as may happen during bereavement. Conversely where a subsequent pregnancy continues without mishap, recent work (Lewis, 1979) suggests that being pregnant may inhibit or delay the full realization and acceptance of grief and mourning. This suggestion is understandable if we consider that pregnancy, psychologically speaking at any rate, is a time of anticipation and looking forward to the future.

Mourning, on the other hand is a time of regret, sadness and searching for that which has been lost in the past. Psychologically, these two states may be difficult to sustain side by side, and it may be that mourning is suspended until such time as the pregnancy is safely over. At that stage, mourning for a parent or previously lost child can be allowed to take place, but a problem may arise where this suspension of grieving 'catches up' with the bereaved, possibly in the early neonatal period when the mother is susceptible to emotional change, 'maternity blues' or post-natal depression.

The consequences of grief and their implications for professionals

As discussed above, the expected consequence is that parents and families will survive the immediate distress of the bereavement, will adapt to the loss, and will make an informed decision, based on facts and information conveyed by health professionals and decide whether or not to embark on a further pregnancy. There will, as indicated, remain a substantial minority, perhaps a third of patients who will have particular difficulties requiring support from another agency (family doctor, health visitor, Public Health nurse, paediatrician, social worker) or one of the self-help groups supporting the bereaved with a similar experience – for example, Compassionate Friends, Stillbirth Association, National Childbirth Trust Miscarriage Groups in the United Kingdom – (similar groups with local chapters exist in the United States).

With intervention these parents too can be expected to adapt ultimately to the loss. But it is helpful, perhaps, for professionals involved to have some guidelines for identifying people with potentially pathological reactions to bereavement, not only in order to identify them and be able to refer them to the appropriate helping agency, for example, psychiatrist, social worker and so on, but also in order that the helper may not unwittingly collude with a pathological process.

Example: One patient referred to above had had a series of neonatal losses from autosomal recessive congenital polycystic kidney disease. In every pregnancy the baby was born but died in the early neonatal period. She had one live child, born 15 years previously and no subsequent successful outcome of pregnancy after 7 or 8 attempts. She was now aged 43. At the time of the last pregnancy it was suggested that early ultrasound investigation might identify an affected baby sufficiently early in pregnancy to allow termination. Conversely, satisfactory evidence that the baby did not have the expected abnormality would allow the pregnancy to go to term. Initial ultrasound investigation suggested that the foetus was not affected, but at a rather unexpectedly late stage a further ultrasound examination indicated that this baby too was affected. In addition to the patient's previous problems and losses, she now had to undergo a mid trimester termination of pregnancy.

Subsequently, it was felt that only the possibility of artificial insemination with the potential of introducing another source of genes, would minimize her chances of continuing to produce babies with this lethal abnormality.

A moment's reflection will suggest that she must have been very determined indeed to achieve a further live baby. Whatever the outcome of such a pregnancy, she would now, of course, require prenatal screening for Down's Syndrome, as well as other hazards of high parity. Because of the confidential nature of the 'treatment' she persuaded the infertility team that AID should be carried out without the knowledge of her family doctor. Subsequently, after a period of months, she came to notice in an emergency when she made a suicidal gesture at the onset of yet another menstrual period, realizing that she had yet again failed to conceive.

Finally, it was felt that AID was no longer likely to have any chance of substantial success and the treatment was stopped. This of course, was extremely distressing for her since as long as it was continued, she could still hope. Since she was not prepared for failure, or even the possibility of failure, this was intolerable.

Forms of pathological mourning

All of the normal stages of grieving can be accentuated – numbness and denial, anger, hostility, self-blame. Grieving or mourning becomes pathological if these normal stages are either excessively prolonged or excessively profound in intensity. It is most important that continuing anger or continuing self-blame should be recognized, appreciated and acted upon.

Sometimes psychiatric opinion, although not necessarily treatment, is required in the management.

Equally important is the observation of various mechanisms of denied or suppressed grief. This may result in the patient who appears to be doing very well, with a particularly 'British stiff upper lip' in its milder forms, but may result in a much more bizarre defensive gaiety in the face of loss, or simply an inability to accept that the baby has died. 'Blocked' grief of this kind can indeed be expressed, given appropriate help, and behavioural methods not requiring medication or necessarily long term psychiatric intervention can be very satisfactory and effective (Mawson *et al.*, 1981).

Chronic grieving, on the other hand, which may persist for an inordinately long period and in addition may be extremely severe in intensity may be more difficult to resolve. In such situations there are usually factors underlying the prolongation of the grieving response which may be partly related to previous personality but is more likely to be related to previous experience of loss for example, or to previous relationships unresolved, or indeed to current life events and problems, which the chronically grieving parent is unable to express or resolve. In this situation, the parent or bereaved person is unable to 'give up' the active grieving for the lost child or baby. Not only does this situation require help, for the relief of the distress caused to the sufferer, but also for the pathological impact which it may have on surviving or subsequent children, and as outlined above on the marital partnership. Where the parent is working, such a syndrome may seriously affect his or her work prospects by producing total preoccupation for most of the time with the loss.

It is sometimes in this situation that well intentioned attempts to suggest that an appropriate period of mourning is now accomplished and the risk of having a further affected child so slight, given appropriate ante natal screening or a statistical calculation of future risk, that a new pregnancy may be embarked upon with confidence. At this stage, the professional may find tremendous resistance on the part of one parent, for example, the mother, which may seem inappropriate or strange, given the very low risk of recurrence or the strong availability of detection prenatally. Such resistance cannot be won over by simple, rational argument and information, since such parents are not by now accessible to rational discussion. Exploration will need to be made either by collaboration with the paediatrician, the family practitioner or social worker or by psychiatric assessment, in order to tease out the contributory factors and also make some treatment strategy for the future.

Grandparents

Other problems may arise when the loss of the first baby, or the news that the baby has been born with a substantial handicap and is unlikely to survive, has given the parents a feeling of guilt or blame. This can, of course, be intensified by grandparents' reaction to a genetically transmitted disorder, for example, a recessive disorder, which arises apparently *de novo* in a family, and much recrimination can ensue.

It may also arise because the parents, when faced with essential information early on in the condition, have been so anxious or so distressed or angry, that they failed to hear the information conveyed. For this reason, whenever it is possible to do so, verbal information and discussion should be backed up with written information which can be digested and discussed, and referred to at home, if necessary more than once, and can be shown to grandparents and friends to improve their understanding.

For example, in the United Kingdom the useful booklet 'The Loss of Your Baby' published by the Health Education Council deals primarily with parents' reaction and questions after a stillbirth, intrauterine or neonatal death. It may be that for parents who have lost a child due to a genetic disorder, individual hospitals or clinics could produce an insert of about one page, each insert covering in outline the main facts about a particular genetic disorder (for example Down's syndrome) which would contain the information which the paediatrician or geneticist wishes to convey to the family on the first or second consultation. This can also form the basis of questions which parents may want to ask at subsequent consultations.

The next child

Although it may seem that the genetic counsellor's task is successfully completed when advice and decisions about a subsequent pregnancy have ultimately resulted in a subsequent child being conceived, carried to term and successfully delivered, this is an over simplification of affairs. It is acknowledged that in the best of circumstances mothers (and fathers) often experience episodic waves of anxiety about the health of the coming child. This natural anxiety is clearly exacerbated by a previous loss, especially when the exclusion of a subsequent affected child, for example neural tube defect, depends on the completion of prenatal screening.

Example: Mrs S. had a routine serum alpha fetoprotein test in a regional screening programme. The resulting level was raised. Recall for a second test was accompanied by an extreme increase in anxiety and at this point in pregnancy her smoking consumption went from 20 to 60 daily and did not return to 20 or below until completion of a satisfactory scan at 20 weeks.

Clearly, anything which can be done to mitigate such an increase in symptoms of anxiety and behaviour which is detrimental to the foetus (e.g. a marked increase in smoking) is worthy of consideration.

An important factor in considering the parents' response is the often voiced self criticism when a mother has previously given birth to a child with a neural tube defect, or other major defect.

Example: Mrs D. had an intrauterine death of an anencephalic baby at 32 weeks. 'For weeks I couldn't bear to look at myself in the mirror. I felt dirty and unclean. I couldn't believe that my body had produced something which the textbooks call a monster'. This sort of statement is not universally voiced by parents, but is fairly common and the underlying feeling (of being disgusted with one's own body) may underline some of the difficulties encountered in helping such patients.

During the next pregnancy it is of course possible that a similar, and detectable, defect may be found and the mother offered therapeutic termination. To some extent, previous experience of the difficulty and the possibility that it may recur is in part preparation, but the sense of loss will recur and should be understood. Many mothers and parents will want to know, provided they can make an informed decision about termination, what effect the event is likely to have on their mental state.

Example: Mrs S. who during the discussions about possible termination for a hitherto unsuspected chromosomal translocation (which was detected unexpectedly, when in fact the defect which was expected was a neural tube defect) was understandably dismayed and distressed at the possible loss of her planned baby. Although very well supported by family, grandparents, friends and a most considerate family doctor, she nevertheless wanted to know in her dilemma what her chances of being depressed or otherwise incapacitated emotionally following the event (the termination) were likely to be.,

Later she talked of her sadness at the loss but emphasized the importance of having accurate information from the counsellor, support from her family regardless of her decision, and time in which to make her decision.

From a statistical point of view it is sometimes helpful to consider the low risk to mental health following termination of pregnancy as discussed in the evidence given to the Lane Report on the workings of the Abortion (United Kingdom) Act 1967 (HMSO, 1974). However, it should be understood that this evidence relates to the most common procedure then available, which was first trimester termination under general anaesthetic. This was, of course, carried out at less than 12 weeks and although often individually sad and distressing at the time, the psychological sequelae, as studied, were minimal provided the individual had a good premorbid history, and was not in other ways vulnerable to depressive or psychotic illness.

In fact, the psychological sequelae of mid-trimester termination of pregnancy are only now beginning to be studied. Clearly, the technology for prenatal screening and mid-trimester prostaglandin termination is relatively recent, and has thus hardly given time to follow up the results and delineate the differences, if any, between first and second trimester foetal loss. It may not be negligible. It can be assumed that there will be some individual differences between loss of an early pregnancy (though as outlined above this in itself may not be negligible), and the planned 'mini labour' form of second trimester termination when the mother may have felt the baby moving and may have seen it on the ultrasound screen.

However, our only hard information at the moment rests on the risk factors available from first trimester termination. It would probably be fair to say that the risk of depression or other emotional upsets is not likely to be less than this and may be perhaps slightly more. On the other hand, however, we do know that preventive measures, good counselling and support, can mitigate the experience of loss and morbidity following on this, so that for any parent who asks the question, one can give a good prognosis with small risk, provided as explained there is no premorbid history of depressive illness. In these circumstances it can be helpful to have advice from a professional experienced in the field.

Where the pregnancy continues, the parents may wish to make frequent contacts with their family doctor or come for medical attention in other ways, because of continuing anxiety. It may not diminish until the subsequent baby is safely delivered. Assuming that the baby is then born perfectly healthy the situation would appear to be simple. However, apart from quite random occurrences of post natal depression it is often difficult for a mother in these circumstances to relate fully to the new baby as wholeheartedly as she would expect. If this occurs, she is likely to feel more guilty than ever, and may become depressed. Usually this situation can be improved by careful support, and guidance. It may be that the birth of such a baby will reawaken feelings of mourning and regret in those mothers who have not adequately grieved for their past losses, but this can often be anticipated by a knowledge of the reaction after the previous infant death. It should be less common if it has been considered in the counselling and management of the bereaved parent in the first place.

More commonly, a baby born following a previous infant loss is of course highly valued and deeply appreciated, and those supporting the family, for example, the doctor and health visitor, will be aware of the possibility of over-protection of this child, particularly where the live child is born after a series of obstetric disasters or losses. It is often assumed that it will be the mother who is very over-protective in these circumstances, but on occasions the mother copes very well indeed, and the over-protection is on the part of the father.

Example: Following the death of a baby at three months, the mother was observed by the health visitor to be dealing very realistically with her loss, expressing her feelings and 'talking through' her sadness and grief, but this was much more difficult for her husband. When, subsequently, they had their second child, the health visitor reported the mother as very competent with the baby and quite relaxed with her once her initial anxiety was allayed. Father, on the other hand, was extremely over anxious about the baby, and indeed the mother found this attitude quite trying and difficult to deal with. By the time the infant was about 12 months old, the mother complained that the father would never let the baby alone in waking hours and was constantly over attentive and over solicitous for its welfare, so that normal development and growing independence was being hampered.

Conversely, where a much longed for and anticipated baby follows a loss or series of losses, complex emotional factors may occasionally result in one or other parent rejecting the child. This is more likely to occur either when, as indicated, the mother's maternal response is inhibited by unresolved grief or depression, or where the lost child was old enough (even where this only has been a matter of months) to have had a definite personality and made its presence known as part of the family. An over idealized view of the lost baby may result in the subsequent baby failing to match expectations and lead to its subsequent rejection.

Practical and administrative aspects

In seeking to minimize the distress felt after an infant loss it is important that attention be given to the parents' needs and wishes at the time regarding funerals and other arrangements such as church services, etc.

For example, until very recently in the United Kingdom, the fact that a stillborn baby was deemed not to have lived resulted in the certification of such a death, not by Death Certificate, but by a distressingly named Certificate of Disposal.

After much effort on the part of concerned paediatricians in Britain, the Department of Health agreed to alter this situation and the Certificate of Stillbirth is now provided by the doctor (no birth certificate is issued), and this must be taken to the Registrar's office within 6 weeks of stillbirth. A Certificate of Burial or Cremation will then be issued to the parents, as for a neonatal death. For babies stillborn before 28 weeks gestation a funeral may be held, but this is not a legal requirement. In addition the parents of a stillborn baby are not eligible for a death grant. The latter is under review by the Department of Health, but at present in any case, this is only £9.00 for babies and intended only to 'offset' funeral expenses. However, the hospital administrators are expected to meet the costs of any stillborn baby's funeral, unless the parents particularly offer to pay for this themselves. This is discussed in some detail in 'The Practical Management of Perinatal Death' (Forrest *et al.*, 1981) where a method for simplifying the administrative procedure can be seen.

The actual arrangements for hospital or private funerals will vary according to locality, and it is extremely helpful if one person in hospital is as familiar with the local procedure as possible. For example, in one large University centre in England, in a very large teaching maternity hospital where there is also a Regional Neonatal Special Care Baby Unit, this responsibility is taken by the Hospital Records Officer, who is very familiar with the procedure and can guide parents accordingly. It has been found to be most important to arrange that more than one person in a department is familiar with the procedure since the system can fail when the usual person is on leave or off sick. Such a person may also take on a very important counselling function. In Oxford, another UK Regional centre, a particular person has been designated as a bereavement welfare officer (the John Radcliffe Hospital, Oxford), and this is similarly a most useful development.

Management

As indicated above the best management of all, sometimes a counsel of perfection, is *prevention*. If adequate support is not given, something like a third to one quarter of unsupported bereaved people may be expected to have further difficulties affecting their physical or mental health. Table 5.2 gives a list of rule of thumb risk factors.

Table 5.2   Bereavement risk factors (after Yorkstone, 1981 with permission)

---

(1) Sudden and unexpected death (as for an unexpected intra-uterine death or sudden death of a neonate not thought previously to be in danger, or an older baby). The death of a handicapped child may cause especial problems
(2) Demands of others causing additional stress
(3) Lack of a close supporting relationship or family member; attempts of family to block grieving after stillbirth or neonatal death
(4) Financial and housing difficulties
(5) No employment outside the home
(6) Known earlier difficulties in dealing with loss or death; evidence of excessive pining, anger or self-reproach
(7) Multiple losses, especially if these have not been adequately acknowledged
(8) Vulnerable pre-morbid personality – previous mental illness or personality inadequacy

---

To this could perhaps be added lack of communication between the parents. This commonly arises out of a desire for one parent to spare the other, but can quickly deteriorate into non-communication, suppressed anger and so on. It also allows unspoken thoughts, fears or blame to reverberate between the parents.

The identification of 'at risk' parents and families must inevitably become a shared task for the family doctor, the paediatrician, genetic counsellor and health visitor. It is difficult to generalize about management since each individual situation and every individual family is unique. However, the principles of prevention, beginning with identification of people at particular risk, should include the capacity to change to a style of counselling more in line with that outlined in the early part of this chapter. This will give the opportunity to disclose particular problems and difficulties and to allow parents to feel that they are able to make decisions on the basis of information, in consultation with the professional, rather than dogmatic instruction.

Appreciation of the normal processes of loss and bereavement and adaptation to them can explain much of the difficulty and resistance commonly encountered, and can enable the professional to give the parents informed reassurance that in the majority of cases these difficulties will diminish in time given adequate support and help.

The manifestations of pathological grieving are as follows:

(1) prolonged grief;
(2) excessive grief;
(3) pronounced and excessive anger, hostility and self blame;
(4) blocked grief or denial, or delayed grieving;
(5) chronic, unresolved grief.

Attention to the features of pathological grieving may identify sufficiently early the parents with special problems who merit specialist referral, opinion and on occasions treatment.

Further, a knowledge of the specialist groups and literature available for bereaved parents is of great value. The case for self-help groups without professional backing is as yet unproved in terms of total preventive care (Parkes, 1980), but undoubtedly for the individual provides the family with information and support which is of benefit and relief to those not pathologically affected, and can be of great immediate consolation.

Counsellors working for Cruse, the British organization supporting the widowed and their families are well aware that, in the words of their Chairman, 'We cannot give to the bereaved the one thing they most want, we cannot call back the lost person. The bereaved know that'. The help from a supportive counsellor or agency or group, however, gives them the confidence that all is not lost. The loss of one person need not undermine trust in all of those who remain.

In this context it seems more than ever important to emphasize that support and counselling, whether from an individual professional or from a self-help group, is a task which creates some degree of 'load' for the counsellor, and if over-involvement or personal stress is to be avoided and the counsellor remain effective, this must be acknowledged and shared. In some professions continuing 'supervision' of the counsellor is mandatory, in order to preserve the counsellor's objectivity and effectiveness. Where the counsellor is not necessarily trained in the inter-personal skills relevant to the task, but is, say, working within a self-help group, it is helpful to plan the support or back-up for consultation about particularly difficult situations in advance. This could be provided as consultation by a professional in a relevant field and need not be an onerous load for the individual consultant.

Other aspects of loss

The birth of a multi-handicapped child

As with other forms of loss and change (for example the adaptation to the amputation of a limb, mastectomy, loss of part of the intestine resulting in a colostomy, loss of a job, loss of status) the birth of a less than perfect child also represents to the parents a profound threat to their 'assumptive world' (Parkes, 1972) and a need to reassess the new situation. Grief, numbness and other symptoms common to other forms of loss have to be worked through with understanding and sensitivity on the part of the professionals involved. Anger (often directed at the doctor or other professional) and hostility must be understood for what they are and not taken personally.

Although it is now common practice to try to help parents by introducing them to a similarly affected child or family, or to a self-help organization which supports sufferers from the condition (e.g. AARG, the Association for Restricted Growth; ASBA, the Association for Spina Bifida and Hydro-cephalus, Down's Association, in the UK), this should be done tactfully and sensitively.

Example: A couple after several childless years had a first baby born with achondroplasia. The mother found great difficulty in accepting, not just the child's handicap but the baby itself. As the mother and baby were being discharged from hospital, in an effort to encourage the mother to bond to the baby and not to reject it, a well-meaning staff member made arrangements to introduce the parents to another family with an affected child. Unfortunately, at a stage when they needed to know the most positive aspects of the condition, they met a family with a much older child who was mentally handicapped as well as short in stature. This introduction, not arranged through the appropriate association, proved disastrous for the mother.

Different problems present themselves where the baby is not only multiply handicapped but the condition is unlikely to be compatible with more than weeks or months of life. Here the parents not only have to face the loss of the 'perfect' expected child, but also have to experience anticipatory grieving in adapting to the future loss. As with grieving and mourning generally, it may be difficult to accomplish anticipatory grieving, which involves withdrawal and introspection, and at the same time function effectively as a parent, spouse, or breadwinner.

Transcultural aspects

Until relatively recently little attention was paid to the effect of culture and ethnic origin on the patient's response to illness and hospital attendance. Clearly however a patient's beliefs, religious practices and customs must affect his or her attitudes to disease, medical and nursing staff and behaviour in the hospital setting

Certain assumptions are sometimes made by professionals as to the effect of belonging to a particular religious group when a death has occurred for example, and insufficient allowance made for the additional effect, on the one hand, of prolonged acculturation in the new country, or recent arrival from a rural environment and village life, on the other.

Hospital staff and other health care workers also need to consider the extent to which they have failed to understand the background, culture and history of migration of particular groups (for example, in England today some groups of immigrants come from very localized rural areas of Pakistan, which may hinder adaptation to life in large cities) (Henley, 1979).

Health service staff can substantially improve services for patients if given relevant information about food prohibitions, washing and toilet customs, naming systems and other practices, for example. They need also to learn effective use of trained interpreters where appropriate (Table 5.3).

In the US, the range of ethnic groups is wider and a useful source of information for staff engaged in practical personal counselling of patients of different origin from their own is now accessible (Marsella and Pedersen, 1981).

Table 5.3   The qualities of a good interpreter (after Cox, 1976 with permission)

Understand both languages well
Be familiar with the psychiatric terms used
Make an easy rapport with both patient and doctor
Be familiar with the cultural background of patient and doctor
Be able to make a linguistic and cultural interpretation
Not be in a hurry

Example: A young mother was observed by the staff of a neonatal nursery to be extremely distressed, weeping and talking of her guilt and unworthiness in the sight of God. She was an Indian girl, reared in Uganda, who had come to Britain to marry without completing secondary education. Her husband, also a Ugandan Asian, was a qualified professional man. Their baby had had some early difficulties and was 'floppy' (hypotonic). During investigation of the baby's neurological problems, a muscle biopsy was performed at a distant medical centre, and the baby stopped breathing during this procedure.

Because of this event, there was uncertainty as to the baby's future, whether it had suffered brain damage and whether it might be handicapped.

The mother's complaints of guilt, self-blame and religious content of her thoughts and speech posed problems of diagnosis for the staff who were unsure of the appropriateness of these in a young Moslem woman, and feared the development of a severe depressive illness in the early post-natal period, made worse perhaps by all the cultural, social and medical stresses she was facing.

A joint approach to diagnosis and treatment, using the intervention and advice of her own Moslem Mullah and assessment by a psychiatrist led to the eventual opinion that a depressive illness was present. She required treatment with anti-depressant medication as she developed strong suicidal feelings before she recovered.

Active support from her religious adviser to the ward staff caring for her, however, and admission to hospital along with her baby (to maintain the attachment) resulted in a satisfactory outcome. In this case, all the sociocultural and ethnic differences, puzzling as they were initially for the nursery staff, had to be considered in the diagnosis and management.

References

Bluglass, K. (1979). Psychiatric Morbidity Following Cot Death. *Practitioner* **224**, 533–539.

Bluglass, K. (1982). Annotation: Psychosocial Aspects of the Sudden Infant Death Syndrome ('Cot Death'). *J. Child Psychol. Psychiat.* **22**, 411–421.

Cox, J. L. (1976). Psychiatric Assessment of the Immigrant Patient. *Br. J. Hosp. Med.* **16**, 38–40.

Forrest, G. C., Claridge, R. S. and Baum, J. D. (1981). Practical Management of Perinatal Death. *Br. Med. J.* **282**, 31–32.

Henley, A. (1979). 'Asian Patients in Hospital and at Home'. King Edward's Hospital Fund, London.

HMSO (1974). Report of the Committee on the Working of the Abortion Act, 1967. Cmnd 5579.

Lewis, E. (1979). Inhibition of Mourning by Pregnancy; Psychopathology and Management. *Br. Med. J.* **2**, 27–28.

Marsella, A. J. and Pedersen, P. B. (1981). 'Cross Cultural Counselling and Psychotherapy'. Pergamon, Oxford.

Mawson, D., Marks, I. M., Ramm, L., and Stern, R. S. (1981). Guided Mourning for Morbid Grief: A Controlled Study. *Br. J. Psychiat.* **138**, 185–193.

Parkes, C. M. (1972). 'Bereavement: Studies of Grief in Adult Life'. Tavistock, London.

Parkes, C. M. (1980). Bereavement Counselling: Does it Work? *Br. Med. J.* **281**, 3–6.

Rutter, M. (1966). Children of Sick Parents: An Environmental and Psychiatric Study. Institute of Psychiatry Maudsley Monographs No. 16. Oxford University Press, London.

The Health Education Council (no date). The Loss of your Baby. 78 New Oxford Street, London WC1A 1AH.

Yorkstone, P. (1981). Risk factors in bereavement. *Br. Med. J.* **282**, 1224–1225.

6 Down's Syndrome

RAY M. ANTLEY
ROBERT G. BRINGLE
KEITH L. KINNEY

Introduction

The goals of genetic counseling are to provide medical and genetic information to help counselees make informed decisions, and to support the counselees as they implement the decisions. These goals are difficult to achieve
because at the time of genetic counseling for Down's syndrome (DS), parents
are experiencing a series of grief reactions related to (1) the shock of the
diagnosis, (2) their perceived change in status emerging from having produced an affected child, and (3) their added financial and physical responsibility. The relationship between the information gained by the parents and their
strong emotional responses changes the character of genetic counseling from
a bland educational activity to an emotionally charged counseling process
that incorporates educational goals (Antley, 1979a, 1979b, 1979c; Kessler,
1979; MacIntyre, 1977).

It is the purpose of this paper to examine the counselees' psychological
responses and to present a plan for accomplishing the goals of genetic
counseling that takes into account the stress reactions of the parents. The
thrust is to provide a practical approach for dealing with psychological and
educational issues when counseling for Down's syndrome.

Psychological reactions of parents – the grieving process

A general model of the grief reaction that provides an understanding of
human adaptation to change can be used to describe a family's psychological
reactions to and acceptance of having a child with Down's syndrome

(CWDS). The model posits that in adapting to change, humans go through a programmed set of identifiable stages designated as shock, denial, anxiety, anger, depression, guilt, bargaining, and acceptance (Antley, 1976; Falek, 1979; Falek and Briton, 1974; Kessler, 1979; McCollum and Silverberg, 1979).

In general, the state of parents of a CWDS is that of persons who have suffered multiple losses or disappointments and who perceive the prospect of continued loss. At stake is the anticipated health and intelligence of their child, and prolonged and expensive dependence of having a CWDS. In addition, the loss and disappointment is heightened by the implication that the counselees may personally be abnormal since they have had an affected child. The intensity of the psychological reactions are directly related to the extent of the perceived loss and to the degree to which the parents value that which has been ruined. Thus, the amount of loss that the counselees perceive can be understood in terms of their knowledge of DS (their perception of the prognosis, recurrence risk, and stigmatization) and the implications of this information for the degree to which their life goals are felt to be threatened. Psychological reactions do not emanate from the loss alone, but occur in the context of the individual's concept of self and the constructs that he or she holds as essential evidence for personhood.

To illustrate the underpinnings of these psychological reactions, one can examine the implication of being genetically defective in the context of a person's and a family's self concept. Prior to the development of a genetic diagnosis, most counselees had not considered that they might be defective. Indeed, the belief in romantic love and marriage in our society leads to couples expecting an ideal family, or at least a normal family. For multiple reasons, expectant parents often look upon their children as self-enhancing extensions of themselves and as sources of status and prestige. Rarely does a couple conceive a child with the knowledge that they are taking a one in twenty risk for a serious birth defect. The disclosure that a child has DS is at variance with prior expectations. With the diagnosis, a new dimension to personal self and family self has to be confronted, one which is perceived as deficient and defective, and for which no previous allowance in self and family concepts had existed. Out of the disappointment, a conflict emerges between idealized self and family, and perceived self and family (Solnit and Stark, 1962). The personal and family adjustment necessary to integrate and bring back into equilibrium the ideal self and the perceived self is the grief process. The resolution of the disappointment or conflict can be viewed as proceeding through the phases previously mentioned, and studies on the psychological aspects of genetic counseling support this thesis (Antley *et al.*, 1973; Antley and Hartlage, 1976).

Shock phase

The shock phase arises when the parents are confronted with the unexpected diagnosis, when they must interact with unfamiliar persons (nurses, consultants, social workers, etc.), and when new information is being introduced (chromosomes, trisomy, ventricular septal defect, etc.). The parents are flooded with stimuli which are suddenly too much to assimilate.

When parents are told they have a child with DS, they usually hear little else. They often become quiet, have surprisingly few questions, and may appear to have understood what was said. Follow-up discussions usually indicate that they heard something was wrong and the rest of the information is either confused or not recalled. The shock phase may last for hours or even days.

Denial-anxiety phase

As the parents begin to reorganize their thoughts following the shock phase, they may or may not acknowledge the possibility that their child has DS. For example, parents will often acknowledge a number of the traits of DS and then explain them away by attributing the palmar creases to one relative, the ears to another, and the Brushfield spots to a third. This behavior can be understood as a tactic to manage their anxiety. The fear of the parents is that if they acknowledge and accept all of the facts, they will become overwhelmed with anxiety and will not be able to cope. Thus, there is a direct relationship between the parents' acknowledgement of abnormality and their feelings of anxiety. As a result, there is a dynamic tension and vacillation between the acknowledgement (requiring anxiety tolerance) and the denial (for anxiety control). As the diagnosis and its consequences are acknowledged they can begin to become integrated into the counselees' reality.

Another source of stress comes from previous attitudes and behavioural patterns of the parents. If the parents had a history prior to the birth of dissociating themselves from and stigmatizing the retarded, the handicapped, and the families of these individuals, then the diagnosis confronts these attitudes and can result in self-stigmatization. The father or mother may also feel they have failed as a spouse by having an affected child. The birth of an affected child is also at variance with previously held expectations for the child and this results in the parents experiencing frustration, anger and depression. Thus, the emergence of anger, depression and guilt signals a level of cognitive acceptance. Similarly, lack of emotional upset would indicate strong chronic denial and lack of progress in working through the grief response. The process of genetic counseling must follow the grief response so that learning can continue without allowing defenses to be overrun.

Guilt phase

A consistent finding in the grief response is a feeling of responsibility or guilt. It tends to occur along with feelings of anger and depression during the period when denial is lessening. There is a reiterative aspect to guilt in which the person repeatedly goes over the events leading to the diagnosis. In a healthy sense, guilt can be seen as an attempt to hold on to the previously held hopes for a normal child while indicating some acceptance of abnormality in the CWDS. The state of being the parent of a normal child compared to that of being the parent of a CWDS appears to be in such sharp contrast that the parental identity before diagnosis seems disconnected from that after diagnosis. The process of working through guilt can be understood as helping the grieving person integrate these two disparate identities and dealing with the accompanying feelings.

Thus, guilt indicates an acceptance by the parents of some limitations of the child, and functions to integrate conflicts within the parental identity. To the extent that it helps to reintegrate the parents' identity, it is part of a normal grieving process. However, guilt, like anger and depression, can be neurotic and become counterproductive to good psychological function if it is chronic and rigid (Smith and Antley, 1979).

Bargaining phase

The bargaining phase usually follows previously described phases and genetic counseling has less influence upon it. Bargaining can be understood as the parents accepting the diagnosis that the child has DS while they are attempting to partially restore the child to normality by making sacrifices. Their hope is to retain a portion of the normal child that they had expected. This, in its more florid form, is seen in the parents saying and/or behaving as if, with sufficient stimulation and training, their child with DS will be restored to a normal learner. Perhaps the more typical response is for the parents to accept the general limitations of DS, but to insist that through extra work their child will be the most advanced in the special education class. Thus, bargaining represents an exchange of work for partial restoration or recovery and has some of the same functions as guilt.

Acceptance phase

The final phase in a resolved grief reaction is acceptance. As acceptance is achieved by the parents, there is a tendency for the denial to disappear and for the emotional upset associated with having a CWDS to subside. Acceptance can be implied by the parents' admission of the disagreeable aspects of having a CWDS and of their inability to change things. Also, a will to change things if the opportunity arises and to adapt to existing circumstances is a positive corollary.

The grief response is a healing response to psychological injury and appears to be biologically programmed. The sudden revelation of the child's having DS is information that raises an implicit question of the parents' worth. During the process of grieving, which in its normal form leads to the restoration of the self-image, the parents usually have to examine their appraisal of themselves and change their values so that they can have adequate self-esteem and be the parents of a retarded child. Genetic counselors need to anticipate and acknowledge these reactions are normal and necessary and genetic education must accommodate to their presence. To understand that these are feelings and responses that persons go through to resolve their disappointment will help counselors be more empathic. This perspective also helps when reassuring parents that their bad feelings are normal. Finally, the grief response and healing aspect of the process are probably best conceptualized as grieving for the self, and its major function is the restoration of the self-concept (Langsley, 1961).

Acceptance of all aspects of DS is not a requisite for successful genetic counseling. On the other hand, genetic counseling which enables parents to make an informed, thoughtful decision requires a level of parental acceptance; therefore, the early stages of the grief process have a direct bearing upon the process of genetic counseling.

Acceptance of the realities of having a CWDS (e.g. long dependency, expensive education, investment of family resources, limited prospect of child's contribution) takes a long time, often more time than professionals appreciate. For example, probably few parents regain psychological equilibrium and acceptance in less than a year. Probably many healthy parents experience significant denial for five years or more. In a sense, gaining acceptance of a CWDS can last for a lifetime since there continue to be new revelations with the passage of time for things which need not or could not have been anticipated.

Thus, parents of a CWDS do not experience a single grief reaction and then return to psychological equilibrium. The experience is better conceptualized as a series of disappointments associated with adjustments that range from the mental retardation of the last child to the need to go through amniocentesis with the next pregnancy (Lippmann-Hand and Fraser, 1979). Because of the multiplicity of demands and the oscillation in responses, it is also instructive to view the parents' psychological responses as a series of crises.

Implications

Some of the implications of the grief response for counseling are that denial and high states of anxiety, anger and depression interfere with learning. The successful handling of the genetic counseling situation depends in part upon the counselors' ability to assess the parents' denial, anxiety, anger, and depression as well as to assess their ability to tolerate these negative feelings. Without accurate assessment and modification of counseling to the counselees' needs, the process may fall short of its goals.

The counselors' understanding of the parental crisis allows them to hold genetic counseling sessions that are planned and focused upon a limited number of well-defined psychological and educational objectives. Furthermore, the identity crisis indicates that the process of genetic counseling challenges the most basic values a person holds and consequently generates great anxiety. This awareness emphasizes the importance of psychological and crisis intervention counseling as a part of genetic counseling. Another implication is that genetic counseling for a new CWDS cannot be adequately provided in a single visit.

Psychological counseling in genetic counseling

The review of the emotional reaction of parents to having a CWDS points out the need for psychological counseling both as a treatment of the emotional impact of having a CWDS and as a facilitator of the genetic education. The advisability of including psychological counseling at the time of genetic counseling suggests a team approach involving a person trained in genetics and another trained in psychological counseling. While one person may be capable of both functions, it is often beneficial to have different persons assume the two roles. Thus, the psychological counselor and geneticist can form a coordinated counseling team. The psychological counselor should be trained in counseling theory and have at least 1000 hours of supervised clinical training. In addition, experience in crisis intervention is important to effective counseling in this situation. In crisis intervention counseling, sensitivity to the dynamics of counselees' defensiveness is acute and the counseling skills to help counselees understand their feelings and to remain open are developed (Reed and Antley, 1976).

Probably the best function of the team is achieved when the psychological counselor is assigned the responsibility for managing the counseling session: making introductions, finding out current counselee problems and questions, validating feelings, controlling the rate at which information is given, and facilitating communication. For example, the psychological counselor may, in the midst of the counseling, halt information being given by the geneticist to attend to the counselees' emotional upset. The purpose of the team approach is to enhance the learning and the degree to which information is incorporated for decision making and to promote the overall healthy adjustment of the parents.

To accomplish this latter objective the psychological counselor can provide additional counseling sessions to promote decision making. The counselor accomplishes this work by (1) helping the counselees understand their feelings and what is causing the feelings; (2) supporting feelings and behaviors that indicate a growing sense of self-esteem; (3) giving support by creating an environment of acceptance, understanding, and concern; (4) helping the parents gain support from each other, relatives and friends; (5) encouraging goal-directed behaviour that is congruent with their values and decisions; (6) attempting to maintain the counselees' continuation of genetic counseling until the task is completed; and (7) providing value clarification (Antley, 1979c; Kinney et al., 1981).

Genetic counseling – general considerations

The foregoing considerations represent the psychological reactions of parents and indicate a need for three different orientations for genetic counseling sessions. They are (1) the informing interview, (2) the supportive counseling sessions, and (3) the counseling and educational sessions. The informing interview is designed to initiate the grief process by providing the parents with the likelihood that this child has DS. The informing interview is held when the diagnosis is suspected and before the chromosome study is complete.

In the discussion regarding genetic counseling that follows, the basic assumptions are that chromosome studies will be carried out on all patients suspected of having DS and that genetic counseling will be performed by a geneticist and a psychological counselor. The chromosome study is recommended for legal, medical, and psychological reasons. It would be a point of potential liability to counsel a family that they have a child with DS when the child does not. The diagnosis based upon physical findings is not error free and the reliability of chromosomes is sufficiently high that they represent the standard of good medical care. Also, it is important to identify translocation carriers. Because of the tenacity of denial in the grief response, it is good psychotherapy to structure the sessions so that parents are initially given tacit permission not to believe the diagnosis. However, when the chromosome results are reported, the focus shifts so that the parents are counseled to accept that the diagnosis is DS. Their denial can then shift to how handicapped the child will be. Thus, the chromosome study is good for the psychological counseling process because it is definitive.

Informing interview

The informing interview is designed to initiate the grief process by providing the parents with the likelihood that this child has DS. The informing interview is held when the diagnosis is suspected and before the chromosome study is complete.

Each counseling session is planned to have a focus; that is, it has a set of issues that coordinates the educational agenda with the counselees' emotional states. Prior to the informing interview an attempt is made to obtain a basic description of the counselees. The medical chart, the referring physician, and nurses can often provide such information as to whether it is the first affected child, whether there is a single parent, or whether a parent has a psychiatric history. Before the informing interview the counseling team should meet to review any such information and to plan the session.

Preparation

The professional participants in the informing interview can assign roles for the geneticist and psychological counselor. Remembering that the counselees' problem will be one of being overwhelmed with stimuli, it is best to keep the number of professionals to a minimum. The confrontation that their child may have DS is the primary issue to be dealt with. The counselors can anticipate that the parents' anxiety will become high and they will probably hear little else. To hold the focus, the counselors can refrain from introducing other issues, particularly those related to descriptions about DS. To decrease the information given at this time, counselees' questions should be answered without elaboration. Asking the parents with whom they plan to share the information helps maintain the focus on the suspected diagnosis. The counselors should encourage discussion of management issues resulting from the situation and avoid discussions on hypothetical, future, or remote situations. For example, a discussion of DS and special education would distract from the primary goal of the informing interview and would cause more anxiety than necessary. The parents' consideration of whom they will tell and how they might tell them is beneficial to their preparation for learning the results of the chromosome study. Effort should be made to maintain the informational focus as a therapeutic objective; specifically, the reality that DS is suspected. The psychological focus can be upon the parents' sadness. Empathy, understanding, and acceptance of counselees' feelings of shock and denial are appropriate therapeutic responses from the counselors. If the informational focus is not held, then the parents' psychological needs may not receive sufficient attention (Antley and Hwang, 1977).

Awareness that a child may have DS usually comes either in the nursery or at a well-baby checkup. In either case, the informing interview should be delayed until the father is present. When this is not done, the mother, especially on the delivery unit, will often frantically try to reach and inform the father by 'phone. Informing the parents separately increases the difficulty of the parents in being mutually supportive to one another. If this cannot be done, we recommend telling the father first, and then the mother.

The session

In the informing interview the counselors are new to the parents and introductions are necessary. Next, it is helpful to ask the parents what they have been told and have observed themselves. How they answer these questions guides the counselors as to where to begin in the informing interview. The parents can be told that Down's syndrome is suspected, emphasizing that the diagnosis is only suspected. On the first encounter, it is not necessary to give a likelihood of 100 per cent that their child has DS (Money, 1975). Even a risk of 99 per cent is helpful to the parents by providing them a medically acceptable basis for their denial phase of the grief process. Parents should be told how long the chromosome study will take to complete. The goal of this session is to have the parents accept that the chromosome study needs to be done and the possibility that it may show DS. It is a good idea to have the counselees summarize what they have been told. Before the 15 to 30 minute session ends, a second appointment is arranged.

Evaluation

After each counseling session, it is instructive to assess and critique the session. The counselors should check that they have covered the topics planned. Also the counselors should evaluate the appropriateness with which they communicated empathy, understanding, acceptance, and concern. A tape recording of the session is an effective means for this evaluation.

Supportive counseling session

A second session in one to two weeks should be scheduled to accord with the parents' progress in their grieving. It is important to maintain the relationship and to encourage their continued attention to the suspected diagnosis. A common parental response is to discuss the problem as little as possible. This requires intervention because it indicates that their primary coping pattern is denial. The overuse of denial has deleterious effects because it signals an arrest in their progression through the grief process. Secondly, this pattern inhibits the parents' communication and mutual support. Each parent may think the other is unconcerned and uncaring because there is little discussion. Also, the denial cannot totally suppress the feelings of grief and the more demonstrative parent may begin to feel he or she is abnormal for being emotionally upset. The purpose of the supportive counseling session is to assess each of these areas and to provide psychological counseling where indicated. This session can often help parents cope better and feel better. When the counselors have been helpful at this session, trust and rapport are built.

Preparation

Knowledge from the informing interview and subsequent contacts by telephone, and information from the referring physician, social worker, and nurses provide a basis for anticipating the counselees' responses at the next session. The anticipated responses tend to fall into a pattern of (1) telling no one and not discussing the diagnosis, (2) discussing the possibility of the child having DS and sharing the news with a few trusted friends, or (3) discussing the problem with everyone but reporting that no one is providing any help. Based upon the information collected, it is often possible to predict the type of counseling session. This anticipation by the counselors can help them prepare their therapeutic responses and to be more accepting of the counselees' feelings.

It is important to time this session so that it occurs before the chromosome study is complete. If this is not done, then the focus of the session is shifted from the parents' grief to the genetic information. From a counseling perspective, having this session occur prior to the chromosome results is a propitious opportunity to provide psychological counseling because it can be oriented to emotional reactions and concerns before the confrontation of new genetic information.

The session

An hour should be reserved for this session. The session is started with open-ended questions regarding what has happened to them since the last visit. Usually there are a number of questions about DS. Often the questions are raised by the parents in an attempt to evaluate the validity of the diagnosis.

Before the chromosome study is complete, the parents usually maintain their hope that the child will be normal. Every effort should be made on this visit to avoid confrontation by the parents that the child has DS. If asked, the counselor can reply that the probability is 70 to 90 per cent. After answering the questions, the counselors need to refocus the session on the parents' adjustment since the birth, the nature of communication that has existed, and what sources of support the family has had. This psychologically-oriented session provides grief counseling for the parents and gives the counselors an opportunity to know the counselees. If the parents ask questions which anticipate that the child has DS, it is a good idea to suggest the question be covered next time if the chromosomes show DS. If the counselor begins to give genetic information, it should be done with the objective of keeping their anxiety level low enough so that they can function, but high enough that they return for additional counseling. This is an example of how the counselors can work to hold the focus of this session on the parents accepting the possibility of the diagnosis and upon the parents' psychological distress (Kinney and Antley, 1976). At the conclusion of the session, an appointment is made for reporting the chromosome results. If the parents are open to an additional appointment before the chromosome results are completed, it can be scheduled with the psychological counselor.

Evaluation

After this session, the counselors' evaluation includes an assessment of how far the counselees have progressed in the grief process. Also, the counselors can evaluate their thoroughness and the quality of their psychological counseling skills. Finally, the information about the counselees that has been gained in this session is of importance in planning future genetic education and psychological counseling sessions.

Genetic education and counseling

The purpose of this phase is to provide the family with the genetic information about DS and with the psychological counseling required to prepare them for making informed and thoughtful decisions. Ideally, this is accomplished in a series of visits about two weeks apart. Information presented will include the chromosome results, the developmental and medical expectations for a person with DS, and the treatments. Having specific objectives in planning these sessions improves the educational activities and counseling process. For example, in genetic counseling some of the information that the counselor gives is contrary to what counselees would like to hear. The disagreeable meaning of this highly personal information affects the processing of the information by the counselees so that either they distort its meaning or are highly selective in their attention. Therefore, it is important to determine whether information is being remembered and integrated for decision making.

Bringle and Antley (1980) have proposed that information available in genetic counseling can be retained by the person in qualitatively distinct ways. At the most primitive level, it is memorized (facts), then it can be conceptualized (understanding), and finally, incorporated for decision making (personalization). Personalization calls for the generalizations and conceptualizations of the understanding phase to be extended so that they apply to the counselees' own life situation.

The three levels of information (facts, understanding, and personalization) are hierarchically related; that is, facts are necessary prior to concept formation and understanding. In a similar manner, general understanding precedes specific applications in personalization. All of the information is not equally valuable for informed decision making. The more specific the understanding (personalization) relative to the particular situation (counselee decision-making), the more likely it is to be used in decision making.

In evaluating the counselee's progress during genetic counseling, the counselor can assess whether, for example, the counselee can remember nothing (i.e. no facts), or can recall isolated bits of information but demonstrate no overall understanding of how they go together. This evaluation, in turn, is carried out across the topics of interest: diagnosis, prognosis, recurrence risk, and options. Table 6.1 illustrates how this evaluation would work for DS. Before each counseling session, the counselor can assess where the counselees are in relation to their integration of the genetic information, and plan the educational objectives accordingly. The focus each time is to move the counselees towards personalization of each of the respective content areas.

The learning and incorporation of the genetic information relates to the psychological reactions of counselees. It is the genetic information and its meaning to the individual that causes the psychological reaction seen in parents of CWDS. This implies that there is no 'diplomatic' way in which the counselees can be told the diagnosis without experiencing emotional upset. Similarly, the counselees' success in personalizing the genetic information provides an estimate of their progress towards psychological acceptance of the situation.

In addition to the genetic information concerning DS, the personality of the parents and the characteristics of their relationship are psychological aspects that must be attended to and incorporated in genetic counseling. A

Table 6.1   Integrating genetic content with the learning model

	Diagnosis	Prognosis	Risk	Options
Facts	Down's syndrome has an extra chromosome	30% of children with DS have Congenital Heart Disease (CHD)	The recurrence risk is 1–2%	The options are as follows: (a) take risk, (b) prenatal diagnosis, (c) adoption, etc.
Understanding	Trisomy leads to cascading effect of multiple congenital abnormalities and mental retardation	Children with DS may die early in life	One or two couples out of every 100 with one CWDS will have another in their next pregnancy	Couples can choose to exercise options in the following way. . . .
Personalization	My child with DS may have MR	My child with DS may have CHD and may die in early life	In *our* next pregnancy the chances of a recurrence is 1–2 in 100	We have the following choices to make in our own life. . . .

basic psychological interview by the counselor is carried out to develop psychological profiles which include evaluating counselees with regard to serious psychological disorders, marital conflicts, determining their sources of emotional support, assessing their present emotional upset, and evaluating their communication skills. The psychological assessment is planned to identify information that was missing in previous sessions.

In some cases, patients present themselves for genetic counseling for the first time with the chromosome study complete. In this circumstance, the psychological interview takes on more importance because it may be the only source of information and provide the only opportunity to build rapport before the major confrontation of the chromosome results. Antley (1979a) has described a method for this assessment that can be used when counseling is provided by a nonpsychologist.

Preparation

Planning the third session differs from the previous two because the chromosome study has confirmed the diagnosis. The confirmation of the diagnosis begins to push the parents to give up their old hopes for a child with normal intelligence, and again will stimulate parental defenses and anxiety.

At the meeting of the clinical personnel, the duties of the counseling session are assigned. A preliminary assessment of the counselees' knowledge and emotional state are made. Also, an estimate of the level of the parents' acceptance is instructive for beginning the session and for planning the pace of the session. The focus for the forthcoming session is to confirm the diagnosis and answer questions. The discussion can usually be guided towards the more immediate implications of the diagnosis and the parents' anxiety. The educational objectives can be conceptualized in terms of facts, understanding, and personalization of the content areas that are to be covered. Usually the diagnosis, the child's developmental expectations, and the recurrence risk are the content areas for the first of these sessions. In subsequent sessions, this information can be reviewed, and prenatal diagnosis and other content areas can be introduced and discussed. Ideally, the objectives will be specific and can serve as a basis for evaluation (Seidenfeld *et al.*, 1980).

The session

The first task in this session, even before the chromosome results are presented, is to obtain a psychosocial assessment. The psychological counselor can use this phase of the session to be supportive to the parents while interviewing them. Also, the insights gained help appraise the counseling team of the parents' level of upset. Finally, the rapport the psychological counselor gains is used during the rest of the session to facilitate communication of the genetic information and its understanding and personalization. Between this initial interview and the session proper, the counseling team can meet again for last minute planning dictated by what the psychological counselor has learned in the psychosocial assessment.

In this session, and each of the subsequent sessions, it is usually beneficial to determine what the parents know and how they have been managing (Antley, 1977). This can be followed by asking what they hope to learn at this session. Their answer to this last question indicates their psychological preparedness to hear the results of the chromosome study later in the session. The counselor attempts to exert control over the rate at which information is given to counselees. The rate of giving information needs to be geared to the counselees' preparedness to learn and integrate the information. Usually, the gradual learning of the diagnosis is best. It is both deleterious to the parents' emotional state, and counterproductive to the learning process, if too much information is given, or if the information is given too rapidly. It is the job of the counselor to slow down the process and to set a rate that does not exceed the counselees' coping abilities.

After providing genetic information, counselees are asked to review their understanding of the information. This review improves learning, identifies deficiencies, and helps the counselors assess the parents' anxiety. For example, if they cannot recall the information or are confused, then their anxiety is probably high and giving information should be halted (Money, 1975). At this point, the psychological counselor would explore with the counselees their emotional upset. If the counselees will talk about their emotional upset and the information that has caused them distress, then their anxiety will usually lessen, and giving information can resume. Alternating between the process of giving information and attending to anxiety, management develops into an effective rhythm for the psychologist and geneticist (Kinney and Antley, 1976).

These sessions are continued until the prognosis, recurrence risk, options for dealing with the risk, and prenatal diagnosis are covered. The subsequent visits may have less involvement of the geneticist and more of the psychological counselor. During these visits the psychological counselor can review genetic information using audio-visual presentations. The counselor helps the counselees in evaluating their genetic risk, their desire for an additional child, birth control, sterilization, prenatal diagnosis, and termination of a pregnancy. Strong evidence for personalization and their capacity to engage in informed decision-making is obtained by having them rehearse their decision making with the psychological counselor.

Often counselees will have two values they hold which they have never before had to choose between. For example, people often have a value not to have an abortion. Also, most couples with a genetic risk for a retarded child have a value to avoid this occurrence. In value clarification, the psychological counselor helps the individual sort out which of any two values, that may be in conflict, has the greater value. Then the counselor helps the couple evaluate whether they are in agreement. If they are not in agreement, then the counselor may need to advocate additional counseling for the purpose of helping them reach a decision. Genetic counseling that continues until the management decisions are openly discussed usually marks a successful completion of the task. The 'right decision' for any particular counselee may be to take a risk. A primary purpose of genetic counseling is to promote informed, thoughtful decision making.

Following the session, a letter to the parents summarizing the information covered is a useful form of documentation (Hsia, 1974). Also, the written record provides a source to which the counselee can return for accurate information at a future time. Finally, it provides the genetic counseling team with documentation of what was covered in the session in case medical or legal questions arise.

Evaluation

Evaluation follows each genetic education and counseling session. Determination of counselees' understanding of DS can be based upon observations made during the session or by objective measurement of the degree to which facts were retained and if understanding and personalization were reached (Antley and Seidenfeld, 1978; Braitman and Antley, 1978). Where the objectives were not met, the sessions should be evaluated as to whether the counselees' anxiety was misjudged, the rate of information was inappropriate for the situation, or the counselors' responses lacked sensitivity to the emotional state of the counselees. Also, the session can be evaluated to determine if the family is progressing through the grief process and whether or not more intense psychological counseling is to be recommended.

By the end of these multiple visits, the family should have evolved through the shock phase and be making significant progress towards a new and altered identity that includes being the parent of a CWDS. This is not always the case. Some counselees and families never integrate the experience and fail to regain their self-esteem. It is helpful to recognize this and to encourage counselees who have difficulty with self-esteem to continue in psychological counseling. One way of thinking about the degree to which the identity crisis is resolved is to ask the question, 'Has the counselee incorporated the fact that they are the parents of a child with mental retardation, Down's syndrome, and do they believe and behave as if they are good people, i.e. have they resolved their guilt, claimed that they are a worthy spouse, and feel that they are an asset to the community?' If counselees report they are concerned that they are having bad feelings about their self-worth, this is reliable information to which the counselor can respond. However, the converse is not true. Reports of good self-esteem (e.g. reports of not feeling guilty) are not sufficient evidence that the crisis is resolved. The counselees' behavior is a better guide. Behavior that can be used as evidence includes the following: overprotectiveness of the child suggests guilt; passivity in marital relationships should raise questions about the person's security and feelings of worthiness in the marriage; overzealous activities to change society with regard to mental retardation should be evaluated for possible reaction formation; and defensiveness specific to DS may be a clue to an exaggerated insecurity and reflect important self-esteem issues.

Counselees do not always follow medical advice, especially in seeking psychological counseling. For counselees to use genetic counseling effectively requires a high level of maturity and psychological functioning. Not all counselees will be this mature and others who are will be so upset by the assault upon their self-esteem that they will not be making good decisions and acting upon them. When this happens, no matter how skilful the counseling, genetic counselors will have only limited success. Primary physicians can be crucial in supporting the families as they attempt to manage their affairs. Specifically, the family physician can encourage the family to continue genetic and psychological counseling.

Although psychological counseling is the best treatment for those who are impulsive and have immature personalities, time does help those who have basically good mental health. Thus, to spread out the counseling over several visits tends to improve the overall success by allowing more time for adjustment.

The evaluation needs to be balanced between a serious critique of the counselors' success in carrying out the plan for the sessions and an appraisal of the counselees' willingness and ability to make high quality decisions. The goal of the evaluation is for the counselors to understand the reasons the counseling progressed as it did and to accept the intrinsic limitations of a process that depends upon good psychological functioning of the counselees for success to be realized.

Conclusions

Genetic counseling is often the only medical intervention in a newborn with DS that addresses the fundamental issues of guilt, responsibility, parental self-esteem, and longer-term implications. The genetic understanding emerging from the chromosome results is initially frightening to the parents, but this knowledge also offers them a rational, physical explanation for what has happened. This knowledge has the potential for focusing their diffuse and unproductive anxiety into activities that deal with the management of the problem. Through this process the parents can begin to gain control over the problems associated with having a CWDS.

Furthermore, the process of obtaining information in genetic counseling sessions provides parents with vocabulary and concepts to explain DS and its implications to others. This is important as they recruit support from other family members and friends. Also, the ability of the parents to continue in normal relationships with relatives and friends is therapeutic because it helps to assuage their guilt and to maintain their self-esteem. Not all of the benefits of genetic counseling for DS are psychological because the knowledge gained provides the parents with background information for making decisions about medical treatments and future child bearing.

Thus, the genetic counselor has an opportunity to deal with parents in the early stage of a life crisis. Genetic counseling can be crucial in guiding the family towards a healthy adjustment rather than allowing them to flounder in their confusion and grief. Also, there are larger social concerns implicit in providing effective genetic counseling for DS and other genetic diseases. In recent years there has been a change in the way geneticists view genetic counseling. This is based upon studies and clinical experiences that indicate that many counselees fail to retain the information about diagnosis and recurrence risk and suffer acute emotional reactions at genetic counseling. This awareness among geneticists is probably best demonstrated in the definition of genetic counseling (Fraser, 1974) adopted by the *Ad Hoc* Committee of the American Society of Human Genetics (1975).

Approaches to genetic counseling that deal with the full range of counselees' problems are of broad social importance because they make technological advances more beneficial for parents and their families. For example, in DS, the knowledge of prenatal diagnosis means that the family can choose to complete their family size without risk of recurrence.

Alternatively, ineffective approaches to genetic counseling create a disparity between the technological capability to improve the quality of human reproduction and the lack of knowledge of these options by those with affected children. Educational background and social class interact to accentuate this disparity. Findings which indicate that many counselees do not retain information provided in genetic counseling can be used to support the argument that many counselees are not capable of making responsible decisions. However, the other side of the argument is that such a conclusion is premature, and that the emphasis on the technological developments in genetics is not balanced with a reasonable effort to deal with the grief of the counselees so that they can personalize the information and make informed decisions. This position also shifts the responsibility for shortcomings in the outcome of genetic counseling from the counselee to the counselor. A responsive commitment to deal with this issue of the potential effectiveness of counseling will reduce the disparity between technology and the scientific literacy of the public, maintain public confidence in genetics, and increase the likelihood of informed decisions.

Acknowledgement

This work is supported by the Department of Medical Research, Methodist Hospital of Indiana. The authors wish to thank Mary Ann Antley, Marla Contz MD, David Weaver MD, and Joe C. Christian MD for their comments on the paper.

References

Ad Hoc Committee on Genetic Counseling (1975). *Am. J. Hum. Genet.* **27**, 240–242.

Antley, M. A., Antley, R. M. and Hartlagê, L. C. (1973). Effects of genetic counseling on parental self concepts. *J. Psychol.* **83**, 335–338.

Antley, R. M. (1976). Variables in the outcome of genetic counseling. *Soc. Biol.* **32**, 108–115.

Antley, R. M. (1977). Factors influencing mother's responses to genetic counseling for Down syndrome. In 'Genetic Counseling' (H. A. Lubs and F. de la Cruz, Eds), pp. 97–108. Raven Press, New York.

Antley, R. M. (1979a). Genetic counseling for parents of a baby with Down's syndrome. In 'Genetic Counseling: Psychological Dimensions' (S. Kessler, Ed.), pp. 115–134. Academic Press, New York.

Antley, R. M. (1979b). Genetic counseling: problems of sociological research in evaluating the quality of counselee decision making. Am. J. Med. Genet. 4, 1–4.

Antley, R. M. (1979c). The genetic counselor as facilitator of the counselee's decision process. Birth Defects 15, 137–168.

Antley, R. M. and Hartlage, L. C. (1976). Psychological responses to genetic counseling for Down syndrome. Clin. Genet. 9, 257–265.

Antley, R. M. and Hwang, D. S. (1977). The Down syndrome – modern genetic counseling. Continuing Education, 56–64.

Antley, R. M. and Seidenfeld, M. J. (1978). A detailed description of mothers' knowledge before genetic counseling for Down syndrome, Part I. Am. J. Med. Genet. 2, 357–364.

Braitman, A. and Antley, R. M. (1978). Development of instruments to measure counselee's knowledge of Down syndrome. Clin. Genet. 13, 25–36.

Bringle, R. G. and Antley, R. M. (1980). Elaboration of the definition of genetic counseling into a model for counselee decision making. Soc. Biol. 27, 304–318.

Falek, A. (1979). Use of the coping process to achieve psychological homeostasis in genetic counseling. In 'Genetic Counseling' (H. A. Lubs and F. de la Cruz, Eds), pp. 179–188. Raven Press, New York.

Falek, A. and Britton, S. (1974). Phases in coping: the hypothesis and its implication. Soc. Biol. 21, 1–7.

Fraser, F. C. (1974). Genetic counseling. Am. J. Hum. Genet. 26, 636–659.

Hsia, Y. E. (1974). Parental reactions to genetic counseling. Contemp. Ob/Gyn. 4, 99–106.

Kessler, S. (1979). The psychological foundations of genetic counseling. In 'Genetic Counseling: Psychological Dimensions' (S. Kessler, Ed.), pp. 17–34. Academic Press, New York.

Kinney, K. and Antley, R. M. (1976). Balancing information giving and anxiety control. Excerpta Med. Int. Congr. Ser. 397, 84.

Kinney, K., Reed, K. E. and Antley, R. M. (1981). Genetic counseling: new opportunities. Bull. Am. Protestant Hosp. Assoc. 44, 20–25.

Langsley, D. G. (1961). Psychology of a doomed family. Am. J. Psychother. 15, 531–538.

Lippman-Hand, A. and Fraser, F. C. (1979). Genetic counseling: provision and reception of information. Am. J. Med. Genet. 3, 113–127.

McCollum, A. T. and Silverberg, R. L. (1979). Psychological advocacy in counseling. In 'Counseling in genetics' (Y. E. Hsia, K. Hirschhorn, R. L. Silverberg and L. Godmilow, Eds), pp. 239–260. Alan R. Liss, New York.

MacIntyre, M. N. (1977). Need for supportive therapy for members of a family with a defective child. In 'Genetic Counseling' (H. A. Lubs and F. de la Cruz, Eds), pp. 567–572. Raven Press, New York.

Money, J. (1975). Counseling in genetics and applied behavior genetics. In 'Developmental Human Behavior Genetics' (K. W. Schaie, V. E. Anderson, G. E. McLearn and J. Money, Eds), pp. 151–170. Lexington Books, Lexington, Massachusetts.

Reed, K. E. and Antley, R. M. (1976). Crisis theory: implication for genetic counseling. *Excerpta Med. Int. Congr. Ser.* **397**, 95.

Seidenfeld, M. J., Braitman, A. and Antley, R. M . (1980). The determinants of mothers' knowledge of Down syndrome before genetic counseling: Part II. *Am. J. Med. Genet.* **6**, 9–23.

Smith, R. W. and Antley, R. M. (1979). Anger: a significant obstacle to informed decision making in genetic counseling. *Birth Defects* **15**, 257–260.

Solnit, A. J. and Stark, M. H. (1962). Mourning and the birth of a defective child. *Psychoanal. Study of Child* **16**, 523–537.

7 Mental Handicap

J. A. RAEBURN

Introduction

This chapter is written from a clinical viewpoint and based on the genetic counselling experience I have gained over the past ten years. During that period there have been many new developments, and attitudes, both of the community at large and of doctors, educationalists and other involved professionals, have undergone considerable change. It is virtually certain that the next decade will also see rapid technological developments which will influence and alter public and professional opinions, challenging their basis and ethics. It is an underlying premise of this chapter that, although the genetic counsellor may hold strong opinions about many aspects of mental handicap (MH) and may advocate these publicly, when he undertakes the counselling role in an individual family he must remain impartial and must point out to the family *all* the options they may consider. This distinction, between the doctor's educational role in the community and counselling role with his patients, is essential if the families counselled are to be allowed true freedom of choice. It is important that genetic counsellors are fully aware of their own basic attitudes (and prejudices!), by means of regular interdisciplinary discussions both within and without the specialty of medical genetics.

Severe mental handicap is common in all races and communities, the prevalence in the child population being around 3 or 4 per 1000 (Crawfurd, 1982). There are innumerable causes but specific genetic syndromes, or conditions with a strong familial element, account for at least 25–30 per cent of all mental handicap (Holmes *et al.*, 1972; Angeli and Kirman, 1975; Laxova, Ridler and Bowen-Bravery, 1977; Crawfurd, 1982). However, this must be an underestimate for genetic factors are likely to account for a significant number of those mentally handicapping conditions which are at present undiagnosed (Davison, 1973). Furthermore certain conditions due to environmental causes (e.g. birth trauma due to pelvic disproportion) may

Psychological Aspects Genetic Counselling

recur unless the primary cause is correctly managed. Thus a significant proportion of families with a mentally handicapped child, probably well over 50 per cent, may benefit from counselling. Opitz (1977) has concluded from a study of 1224 patients, in the Central Wisconsin Colony for severe mental retardation, that *all* families with a mentally retarded child should have 'aetiological/genetic counselling'.

If mental handicap occurs on its own or without such serious physical anomalies as major congenital heart disease then, provided adequate physical care is provided, the life span may approach that of normal individuals. This means that the parents may be confronted with the prospect of managing their child's disorder for the duration of their own lives. Clearly considerable professional support must be offered but in the early stages this will be orientated towards making an accurate diagnosis and initiating appropriate specific therapy. However if the doctor's total interest at this stage is directed towards the investigational management of the child, he may forget that this is a time of great uncertainty and insecurity for the parents. Hasty, apparently evasive, answers to anxious questions will leave the parents more anxious and with a developing mistrust of all the professionals involved with their child. In a chronic incapacitating condition such as mental handicap the professional who misleads or confuses the parents in the early stages will demean not only himself but also all his professional colleagues who later try to help the family.

When should genetic counselling be offered?

The answer to this question will obviously depend both on the cause of mental handicap and the time of diagnosis. In the case of Down's syndrome (DS) it was formerly considered that the parents should not be told the diagnosis for some time, often only when they had recognized some abnormality after several months (Keay, 1936). It has been shown more recently, however (Drillien and Wilkinson, 1964; Carr, 1970), that parents of DS babies wish to know the facts about their child's condition as soon as possible. This wish is also usually expressed by the parents of children with other causes of mental handicap, causes which are often not apparent at birth. Furthermore in a small sample of 65 young adults who had no family history of genetic disorder, over 90 per cent said that they would wish genetic counselling, at least prior to marriage, if a genetic disorder had been identified.

The timing chosen by the doctor will also depend on his own reasons for giving genetic counselling. Some of these are classified in Table 7.1. This table emphasizes that the specific genetic reasons for counselling cannot be separated from other aspects of the management. However all these reasons would also rule that counselling should be carried out soon after the diagnosis of mental handicap has been made.

Table 7.1   Major reasons for (genetic) counselling in mental handicap (MH)

---

(1) *Prevention* via:
    (a) family limitation
    (b) prenatal diagnosis and selective termination of pregnancy
    (c) carrier detection in other family members
    (d) elimination of environmental causes of MH

---

(2) *Family support*
    (a) control guilt feelings
    (b) rectify unfounded anxieties
    (c) reassure where appropriate

---

(3) *Lessen extent of handicap*
    (a) reduce deterioration: e.g. special diets or therapy (? bone marrow transplantation in mucopolysaccharidoses)
    (b) institute early treatment for specific difficulties, e.g. speech handicap in the fragile-X syndrome

---

Who should perform genetic counselling?

Many factors will influence the choice of genetic counsellor. There is some controversy, particularly about whether counselling should be done by the diagnosing paediatrician or by a separate genetic counsellor. Whichever approach is chosen there are two important requirements to be met. Firstly, genetic counselling needs a great deal of time and must be organized, for *both* parents, away from a busy out-patient clinic. Secondly, genetic counselling is an integral part of the management of the family and should not be so separate from other aspects that communication between counsellor and paediatrician is impaired. A combined clinic at which the parents discuss the paediatric and genetic aspects with their paediatrician and a medical geneticist respectively will usually be of greatest value and will avoid major contradictions between specialists.

Causes of mental handicap

Mental handicap can be the end-result of many different causative factors either genetic or environmental. There is a considerable excess of mentally handicapped males in most communities, a finding which implicates X-linked genes in aetiology. Recent studies of the fragile X syndromes have added weight to this suggestion. Table 7.2 lists the main aetiological sub-

Table 7.2   Causes of mental handicap (%)

	Holmes et al. (1972)	Regemorter and Raeburn (unpublished)
(1) *Genetic*	*33.5*	*29*
(a) Single gene	(7.0)	(9)
(b) Chromosomal	(19.1)	(6)
(c) Multifactorial	(7.4)	(14)
(2) *Acquired*	*26.4*	*27*
(3) *Mixed or unknown*	*40.1*	*44*

groups and their relative frequencies in mental retardation hospitals based on our own data (Regemorter and Raeburn, unpublished) and that of Holmes *et al.* (1972). The main difference between the two studies is that our own included only patients under the age of 21 years. Thus in that study the number of Down's syndrome (DS) patients, and thence the proportion of MH due to chromosome disorders, was lower since in Scotland younger DS patients are rarely admitted to long-stay hospitals. Since genetic factors may operate in a proportion of the 'unknown cause' group, or must at least be excluded, it is clear that genetic counselling is relevant in the majority of families in which there is mental handicap.

Table 7.3 lists the more common single gene causes of mental handicap; greater details are available in Harper (1981), Bergsma (1979), or, catalogued briefly, in McKusick (1983). In the case of autosomal dominant conditions it could be that there is marked pleiotropy, many different organs being affected variably by the mutant gene. Counselling here requires not only an indication of the genetic risk but also if the child is affected, the likelihood of mental handicap or other medical aspects being severe. In practice a careful compilation of the family tree will usually indicate the extent of such clinical heterogeneity. In addition this pedigree may reveal the true diagnosis by directing attention to the symptoms and signs present in some but not all affected family members. Neurofibromatosis is a good example of a pleiotropic condition with considerable variability in expression. Although mental handicap occurs in rather less than 50 per cent of affected individuals (and an accurate figure is not available) developmental delay is one of the commonest childhood presenting features.

When a healthy couple have a single child who is mentally handicapped either autosomal or X-linked recessive genetic causes must be carefully considered as well as a new mutation to a dominant disorder. Fuller details of all these conditions are available elsewhere (Holmes *et al.*, 1972; Bergsma, 1979) but usually genetic causes can be suspected by noting the presenting

Table 7.3   *Some single gene causes of mental handicap* (proportion with MH in brackets)

---

(1) *Autosomal dominant disorders*
   Tuberous sclerosis (75%)
   Other phakomatoses (e.g. neurofibromatosis) (25%)
   Aperts' syndrome (? is mental handicap preventable)

---

(2) *Autosomal recessive disorders*
   Phenylketonuria (70% if untreated)
   Most forms of mucopolysaccharidosis
   Cerebral lipidoses (50%)
   + many other inborn errors of metabolism
   Severe microcephaly (90%)
   Sjogren–Larsson syndrome (?)

---

(3) *Sex-linked disorders*
   Lesch-Nyhan syndrome (90%)
   Hunter syndrome (50%)
   Non-specific X-linked mental handicap (100%)
   Fragile X chromosome syndrome (see text) (70%)

---

complaint, the age of onset and the pattern of clinical symptoms and signs. Such a check-list will help the doctor to select the most relevant ancillary tests. If an X-linked disorder is likely then careful consideration of the maternal side of the family is essential – an aspect of management which may be omitted if the focus of attention is upon the *diagnosis* of isolated mental handicap in a boy.

Chromosomal causes of mental handicap

A high proportion of unbalanced chromosome anomalies are associated with a severe degree of mental retardation and often too, with severe cardiovascular, renal or skeletal defects. These generalizations apply especially to autosomal anomalies but to some extent they are also relevant in sex chromosome aneuploidies. Table 7.4 lists the different categories of chromosome disorder. It should be noted that apart from trisomy 21 and Turner's syndrome, the numerical chromosome aberrations are almost always lethal, by birth or at least within the first years of life. Structural abnormalities involve much smaller amounts of DNA and longer survival is more likely. Therefore in the mentally handicapped child with multisystem involvement, and often in the parents, careful cytogenetic studies are important. Although it is estimated that many of the undiagnosed mentally handicapping conditions will be due to minor chromosome imbalance, Jacobs *et al.* (1978) found that careful banding studies only identified a small extra proportion of anomalies (2.3 per cent) in a group of 500 in-patients at an MH institution.

Table 7.4   Classification of chromosome disorders causing mental retardation

---

(1) *Numerical disorders*
   (a) Trisomies especially 21, 18, 13
   (b) Monosomy especially Turner's syndrome[a]
   (c) Triple X, quadruple X and other sex chromosome aneuploidies

---

(2) *Structural anomalies*
   (a) Unbalanced reciprocal translocations
   (b) Unbalanced Robertsonian translocations
   (c) Deletions especially of 4, 5, 13, 18
   (d) Fragile X syndrome

---

[a] In Turner's syndrome the IQ is usually normal.

The fragile X syndrome is now a most important chromosomal cause of mental handicap. Recent interest developed after Sutherland *et al.* (1977) had shown that in some X-linked mental retardation families banded chromosome preparations carried out after culturing in tissue culture medium which was deficient in folic acid, had break points present non-randomly on the X chromosomes of affected males and most carrier females. The affected sites were on the long arm (q 27 or q 28) and whereas normal individuals showed this anomaly in less than 1 per cent of cells there was a highly significant increase in affected males to between 5 and 30 per cent. The initial application of these findings was in the potential for carrier detection and prenatal diagnosis within affected families (Jacky *et al.*, 1980). More important still is the possibility that the fragile X chromosome marker will help to diagnose and categorize a major proportion of the families in which there are mentally handicapped males.

Prenatal diagnosis

Some causes of mental handicap can be diagnosed prenatally and the genetic counselling interviews must include an explanation of the procedures involved and the stages of pregnancy at which they are carried out. In general the conditions due to inborn errors or to specific chromosome anomalies can be diagnosed by about 19 weeks gestation following amniocentesis around 15–16 weeks. A major reason for urgency in diagnosing a cause of MH is that, for a particular couple at risk in a subsequent pregnancy, prenatal diagnosis with the option of selective termination of pregnancy may be an important possibility. In a majority of pregnancies monitored in this way the tests will be normal and the couple can then be reassured at as early a stage as possible.

Prenatal diagnosis is an adjunct to the genetic management of these families and will require careful consideration and more counselling time. It is not just a technical procedure which can be embarked on by doctors and scientists without adequate discussion.

Approaches to counselling

The genetic counsellor in mental handicap must have a broad knowledge of the range of conditions likely to cause the disorder and the specific genetic possibilities. The initial interview will identify the extent of handicap in the proband and whether there are any affected relatives. Gathering this information is important in itself but of greater importance is the opportunity it provides for recognizing views and attitudes of the parents (Sensky, 1982; Taylor, 1982). It is much better if both parents of a handicapped child are present at this interview and it is relevant to note how, as a couple, they share out answers to the genetic questions. It is not at all unusual for a couple to be highly critical of the manner in which they were told of their child's handicap or of delays in making the diagnosis. Before accepting such criticisms as completely true, a counsellor should consider the sequence of reactions involved in coping with crises and the possibility that this, rather than a colleague's mistake, accounts for the hostility and possible associated guilt. A counsellor does no good for a family if he reinforces their false allegations against a professional, especially if that colleague is closely involved in the further management. After this type of criticism the counsellor should hear the couple's description of events, along with their feelings of anger, before moving the interview back to genetic topics.

An approach I have found useful in controlling and developing the genetic counselling interview is based on transactional analysis as originally described by Berne (1970). In summary this theory describes any relationship between two individuals, as in the doctor–patient relationship, as a 'transaction'. Each subject can communicate in this transaction at each of three levels as shown diagrammatically in Fig. 7.1. The 'parent' level involves attitudes often established in childhood based on the 'do's and don'ts' laid down then by the parents or other dominant adults. The 'adult' level involves the part of the individual concerned with factual information and data. The 'child' level involves all the emotional reactions. As the figure implies transactions between individuals may be between different levels – for example an emotional client (child) may appeal to the supportive role of the doctor (parent), asking for help in reaching the correct decision. In the figure two different responses are shown.

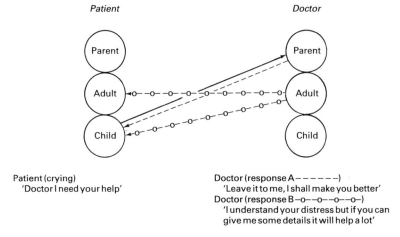

Fig. 7.1   The model of transactional analysis applied to the doctor–patient relationship

Another aspect of transactional analysis relevant in counselling is the suggestion that a contract should be agreed as to the aim of the interview. In genetic counselling this can be achieved by starting the interview with a general enquiry such as 'what are the main questions you wish me to help with?' It is clear that a genetic counsellor aims to provide each couple with information (adult) in an area of great emotion (child) which is sometimes modified by strong prejudices (parent influences). For further information the reader should see Berne (1970, 1975) and Harris (1973).

Resources for the counsellor

Genetic counselling is clearly a highly emotional aspect of the management of a family and it is useful to reinforce the primary interviews by written summaries of the details covered. In some instances there will be books available which give relevant additional information (e.g. Cunningham and Sloper, 1978). This need for suitable reading material has very often been expressed and yet it is only recently that suitable books have been available. Many more are needed. Another resource to be made available to parents of handicapped children would be a list of the agencies available which provide different aspects of support. These are often obtainable as booklets from social work departments.

Many doctors forget that another parent, who also has a mentally handi-capped child, may be invaluable in providing emotional support, especially in the early stages. In addition, it is often stated that for doctors to put such couples in touch with each other is a breach of professional confidence. In my opinion this aspect can quite legitimately be raised, probably at a second counselling interview, and the option of meeting another parent can be arranged if the parents agree. There are now many relevant self-help groups, formed by parents who wish to provide extra support for mentally handicapped persons and their families. Suggesting that a couple might like to make their own contact with such a group allows them to choose for themselves which of the parents, if any, will be able to provide useful support. Although I, at first, tried to choose the most appropriate couples for the consultants to meet, it is better not to control this aspect. Doctors may not always know best, especially in the non-clinical area of emotional support.

Pitfalls in genetic counselling

Many of the most important errors in counselling may be avoided. Of greatest importance is the need to confirm the precise genetic diagnosis and the mode of inheritance. If an accurate diagnosis has not been made then perhaps further investigations are required in both the affected child and the members of the family. If a diagnosis is not possible then the parents must be told so but it is still possible for counselling to be presented in a positive manner (e.g. 'we have not yet been able to make a clear diagnosis but we have excluded virtually all of the conditions with a high recurrence risk' or 'although there is not a precise diagnosis in your child our previous experience shows that the chance of a further child being affected is less than one in . . .').

A major pitfall is for the counsellor to boost his own ego by taking up a directive role and assuming responsibility for the couple's decision. As stated before, his prejudices must be restrained so that the couple reach a decision based on genetic facts and on their own family situation. After they have indicated their decision a counsellor may choose to give his support and he should also detail how best their intentions can be realized and the likely outcomes.

A further problem is when the counsellor is asked a question which he cannot answer. It is too easy to be evasive or to guess or perhaps to answer from a prejudiced viewpoint. It is certain that the parents will eventually find the truth and thus will lose confidence in their counsellor. The best response to unanswerable questions is to admit that one does not know but to promise to try to find an answer.

Finally, a further trap for a genetic counsellor is the articulate couple who forcefully criticize all of the other professionals they have attended. Although it is a temptation to take over, and thus put everything right (!), the counsellor should ask himself whether their hostility stems from their anger that their child is not normal. This couple require more genetic counselling sessions over a longer period than less hostile families. In addition close and tactful co-operation with all the other professionals is essential and is perhaps best secured by arranging joint consultations.

Summary

Genetic counselling for families in which there is mental handicap is not easy. It is essential that a correct diagnosis is reached along with an accurate family history, so that the mode of inheritance can be understood. Failing that, empiric risk figures may be available (Bundey and Carter, 1974). The counsellor must consider the emotional impact of the disorder and of genetic counselling and must make time available on several occasions to answer relevant questions. Other parents of affected children and self-help groups are a vital resource but they must never be forced on unwilling individuals. The genetic counsellor must always work closely with other professional colleagues, so that the genetic management is an integral part of the overall care and support of the family.

References

Angeli, E. and Kirman, B. (1975). Genetic prognosis in severe mental handicap. *J. Ment. Defic. Res.* **19**, 173–193.

Bergsma D. (1979) (Editor). 'Birth Defects Compendium', 2nd edition. The National Foundation – March of Dimes. Macmillan Press, London.

Berne, E. (1970). 'Games People Play'. Penguin Books, London.

Berne, E. (1975). 'What do you say after you say Hello'. Corgi Books, London.

Bundey, S. and Carter, C. O. (1974). Recurrence risks in severe undiagnosed mental deficiency. *J. Ment. Defic. Res.* **18**, 115–134.

Carr, J. (1970). Mongolism: telling the parents. *Dev. Med. Child. Neurol.* **12**, 213–221.

Crawfurd, M. d'A. (1982). Severe mental handicap: pathogenesis, treatment and prevention. *Br. Med. J.* **285**, 762–766.

Cunningham, C. C. (1982). Psychological and educational aspects of handicap. *In* 'Inborn Errors of Metabolism in Humans' (F. Cockburn and R. Gitzelmann, Eds), pp. 237–253, MTP Press Limited, Lancaster.

Cunningham, C. C. and Sloper, P. (1978). 'Helping your Handicapped Baby'. Human Horizons Series, Souvenir Press (E & A) Limited, London.

Davison, B. C. C. (1973). Genetic studies in mental subnormality. *Br. J. Psychiat.* Special publication No. 8, London.

Drillien, C. M. and Wilkinson, E. M. (1964). Mongolism: when should the parents be told. *Br. Med. J.* **5420**, 1306–1307.

Harper, P. S. (1981). 'Practical Genetic Counselling'. John Wright and Son Limited, Bristol.

Harris, T. (1973). 'I'm O.K., You're O.K.' Pan Publishers, Ltd., London.

Holmes, L. B., Moser, H. W., Halldorsson, S., Mack, M. S., Pant, S. S., Matzilevich, B. (1972). 'Mental Retardation: an atlas of diseases with associated physical abnormalities'. The Macmillan Company, New York.

Jacky, P. B., Dill, F. J. (1980). Expression in fibroblast culture of the satellited X chromosome associated with familial sex-linked mental retardation. *Hum. Genet.* **53**, 267–269.

Jacobs, P. A., Matsuura, J. S., Mayer, M. and Newlands, I. M. (1978). A cytogenetic survey of an institution for the mentally retarded: 1. Chromosome abnormalities. *Clin. Genet.* **13**, 37–60.

Keay, A. J. (1936). The infant mongol. *Practitioner* **191**, 173–180.

Laxova, R., Ridler, M. A. C., Bowen-Bravery, M. (1977). An aetiological survey of the severely retarded Hertfordshire children who were born between January 1, 1965 and December 31, 1967. *Am. J. Med. Genet.* **1**, 75–86.

McKusick, V. A. (1983). 'Mendelian Inheritance in Man'. The Johns Hopkins University Press, Baltimore and London.

Opitz, J. M. (1977). Diagnostic/genetic studies in severe mental retardation. *In* 'Genetic Counseling' (H. A. Lubs and F. de la Cruz, Eds), pp. 417–443. Raven Press, New York.

Sensky, T. (1982). Family stigma in congenital physical handicap. *Br. Med. J.* **285**, 1033–1035.

Sutherland, G. R. (1977). Fragile sites on human chromosomes: demonstration of their dependence on the type of tissue culture medium. *Science* **197**, 265–266.

Taylor, D. C. (1982). Counselling the parents of handicapped children. *Br. Med. J.* **284**, 1027–1028.

8 Physical Handicap

IAN PULLEN

Introduction

Physical handicap is a stigma. Not only is it frequently obvious for all to see but the affected person is constantly confronted by his handicap, physically and visually. The odd gait, abnormal posture, walking aid and wheelchair, all signal disability and deficiency, and the stigma will affect all personal interactions (Goffman, 1963).

The impact that physical handicap has on the individual and the family will depend on the nature and extent of the disability, age of onset and prognosis. The birth of a physically abnormal baby may lead to maternal rejection with delayed or defective bonding and permanent impairment of mother–child relationship. The apparently normal little boy who, at the age of 5, is discovered to be suffering from a progressive physical handicap which is life-threatening and for which there is no treatment, presents another set of reactions and problems for the patient and his parents. A further range of difficulties will be encountered by the adolescent or young adult who complains of muscle weakness and is diagnosed as having an inherited condition which is slowly progressive, but is compatible with survival into middle age.

All but the mildest of physical handicaps will affect mobility, body image and relationships with others. The more severe handicaps will interfere with independence, privacy, modesty and sexuality and will dictate where geographically the patient has to live and whether this can be at home or must be an institution.

This chapter will concentrate on the muscular dystrophies because they are relatively common and illustrate well many of the problems associated with physical handicap. They are progressive, genetically determined degenerative disorders of voluntary muscle and are genetically heterogeneous. Many of the types show a similar clinical picture with progressive muscle weakness

Psychological Aspects Genetic Counselling

and wasting, increased serum enzymes and characteristic electro-myographic and histological changes. Different forms however are inherited in different ways and so a precise diagnosis must be made before genetic advice can be given.

Physical disability of early onset

Duchenne Muscular Dystrophy (DMD) is the commonest form of muscular dystrophy and the most severe. It is characterized by progressive muscle wasting and weakness which becomes clinically evident around the age of 3–5 years and leads to an inability to walk by the age of 12 and death in the late teens or early twenties (Emery, 1980). It is inherited as an X-linked recessive trait and only affects boys.

Clinical aspects

At birth, and usually for the first few years of life, the boy appears completely normal. Walking may be delayed beyond 18 months, but he looks physically strong with apparently sturdy calf muscles. Once walking, he tends to waddle, walks on his toes, is unable to run and falls more than his peers and after falling, rises in a characteristic way – 'climbing up himself' with his arms. At this stage, some abnormality is usually evident to the experienced observer – a skilled physician or parent of a previously affected child (Wyngaarden and Smith, 1982).

Unless alerted by a positive family history, it may not be until school entrance that the parents' attention is drawn to the abnormality. He has difficulty keeping up with his classmates, physically and sometimes academ-ically because there is frequently an associated non-progressive mental retardation. A survey of 38 DMD boys demonstrated a mean IQ of 83. Their normal siblings had a significantly different mean IQ of 110 (Vignos, 1975). Growth and increased co-ordination can compensate temporarily for the concurrent progressive weakness and wasting, but inevitably further signs of progression soon emerge. Weakness starts proximally, affecting trunk mus-cles with increased lordosis and protuberant abdomen. Walking up slopes and stairs requires help; then arms become weak so that he has difficulty dressing, undressing and toileting.

Management should be directed towards achievement of positive goals: he should be helped to lead as normal a life as possible, physically, socially, emotionally and intellectually (Vignos, 1975). He can generally attend the normal local school while ambulant. When walking becomes unsafe, is only possible with detrimental stress on the upper limbs, or is physically exhausting (Bossingham *et al.*, 1977), usually between the age of 11 and 13, he ceases to walk and requires a wheelchair. Independent ambulation should be maintained for as long a time as is reasonably possible as it is suspected that premature confinement may result in unexpected and undesirable side-effects including accelerated physical and psychological deterioration (Vignos, 1975). However, this should not be carried to extremes. For example, one centre tried to keep boys walking in long leg braces after they had 'gone off their feet' and succeeded to the point of keeping them walking for a further two or more years, 'but only at the cost of missing a great deal of schooling and social contact with other people, which . . . might perhaps have been more important' (Gardner-Medwin, 1975).

Contractures appear, at first affecting the feet, but once he stops walking flexion contractures limit movement of knees and scoliosis is a problem of prolonged sitting. Braces may be needed to keep him upright in his chair and night splints and physiotherapy may minimize restricted joint movement. At one time, extensive surgical procedures were advocated to correct the flexion deformities but now in many centres there is a swing towards minimal intervention with surgery limited to tendon lengthening procedures. Decreased physical activity commonly leads to obesity which requires dietary advice as it makes lifting, cleaning and balance more difficult.

Once confined to a wheelchair, the normal school may be unable to cope in which case transfer to a special school will be needed. Most parents prefer a day school with other handicapped children rather than an institution a long way from home (Zellweger, 1975).

As the muscle weakness progresses life becomes increasingly restricted. He will be able to do less and less for himself and in addition to being washed, dressed, toileted and fed, in bed at night he will need to be turned regularly because of leg pains and to avoid the development of pressure sores. Hard-pressed and tired parents may also have to cope with incontinence. Respiratory excursion decreases leading to increased susceptibility to chest infection which, coupled with cardiac involvement, eventually leads to death in the late teens or early twenties.

Social aspects

Any chronic disabling disease has considerable impact on the whole family (Zellweger, 1975). The major social effect of a boy developing DMD is some degree of isolation for the whole family. This may be a withdrawal by the family itself, but may also be the response of relatives, neighbours and friends who tend to pity, ignore or actively avoid the family.

There is a perpetual restriction on the family's freedom and activities, particularly if they are reliant on public transport. The young DMD boy can be carried on to buses and trains and into cars but eventually becomes too heavy for this to be possible. The home will have to be modified with ramps and other aids and a move to ground-floor accommodation may be necessary.

Handicap proves to be a considerable burden. In Britain, the Department of Health and Social Security will provide an indoor electric wheelchair but not an outdoor model. Thus, a family may find it difficult to obtain an outdoor chair and a power hoist to enable the chair to be transferred to a van. An electric hoist can make bathing easier and electric beds simplify turning at night.

Above all, the daily routine is disrupted and parents progressively have to do more for the child in the way of delivering and collecting him from school, dressing and toileting at the stage where the parents of normal children are being relieved of these tasks. While at home, the DMD child will require someone always to be in attendance. The family will become involved with a large number of professionals, including paediatricians, general practitioners, geneticists, orthopaedic surgeons, health visitors and social workers, and will spend a considerable amount of time visiting hospital clinics. A report by the Muscular Dystrophy Group of Great Britain has recommended better co-ordination of professional help.

Emotional aspects

The patient

Symptoms rather than the notion of disease *per se* often have a profound impact on the affected child's emotional development (Fischman, 1979). In the early stages, he is not consciously aware of any difference between himself and other boys. Later, he may try to over-compensate for his weakness by pushing himself to his physical limits with consequent exhaustion, and symptoms lead to such questions as, 'Why can't I run like other boys?'. Characteristically, however, these symptoms often provoke few questions from the boy about his illness. In some cases, this may be due to the related mental deficiency and especially poor verbal ability.

Recognition that his peers are both physically and sometimes intellectually his superiors may lead to avoidance, withdrawal and depression. Increasing dependence at a time when he should be gaining independence, precludes an easy transition through adolescence (Fischman, 1979). Some children will have difficulty with parents who are over-protective and may become very angry with them and actively resist their help.

Giving up walking will be another major hurdle for the DMD boy. Temporarily there may some relief, but soon the electric chair will lose its novelty and it will be some time before 'the wheelchair is seen as a symbol of mobility rather than invalidity' (Nichols, 1971).

Modesty and personal privacy are compromised when the DMD child becomes totally reliant on someone else to wash and clean him, help him micturate and clean him after defaecation. This physical closeness may make the discussion of sexual matters even more difficult than in the normal family. How does the developing adolescent cope with the normal experimentation with sex when he may be too weak to masturbate and is socially isolated? Parents tend to avoid enquiring about sex and make their observations from a distance. When questioned directly, frequent responses are 'I don't think it troubles him' or 'I've seen no sign of any problem'. Professionals may avoid discussing the subject with adolescents ostensibly for fear of causing them distress. The few systematic enquiries that have been reported are conflicting. 'Nobody ever talks about the sex life of these adolescent muscular dystrophy children . . . I gathered that want of sexual activity, including inability to masturbate, appears not to be a cause of frustration' (Zellweger, 1975).

Morgan (1975) reporting group discussions with DMD boys – 'There was a uniform denial that sexual deprivation was a cause of distress to them. They described sexual fantasies about young women with whom they had formed attachments but did not seem to want these fantasies to be translated into reality'. However, Staples (1977) had no doubt 'that some boys do find problems of sexual expression extremely distressing and can see no solution', and Bayrakal (1975), reporting a group experience with adolescents with muscular dystrophy, states 'The vicarious gratification of talking about romance and sex was not enough. David (a member of the group) said, "What is left for the cripple but to grab your dinkie and play with it". Carlos responded immediately by saying, "I can't even have that. I can't reach that bloody thing".'

There is a very close correlation between body image and self concept (Schechter, 1960). We look to see if other people approve or disapprove of us in our activities, dress and appearance. A normal critical developmental task in adolescence is the reformation and consolidation of the person's body image. Common strategies for coping are avoidance and over-compensation. Social withdrawal, loneliness and depression become worse as the condition progresses. Most boys slowly withdraw from contact with others including family members. They look depressed and apathetic, speaking little and seldom initiating any activity. 'The feeling of hopelessness for the future is strongest in adolescence when the impact of their lack of attractiveness and the unrealistic conceptions they've maintained about cure and job future really hits' (Schechter, 1961).

Some parents allow their children to believe that they will get better in the future. Buchanan *et al.* (1979) found that 6 out of 25 affected boys had not been told they had muscular dystrophy. They were aware that they were 'different' from their peers, with a sense that the weakness was something within their control, that is, the result of their own incompetence. The other 19 boys had been told some of the details regarding their disability. The usual explanation was that they had 'weak muscles'. Only one boy, aged 14, knew that he had a terminal illness and tended to be withdrawn and depressed. Staples (1977) found that in contrast to problems with sexual matters, the boys appeared to manage the concepts of premature death without disquiet. Certainly, while attending a special school, they become increasingly aware of the death of other children. 'Indeed, one has heard stories of these children in schools who, in early adolescence, place bets as to who will be "the next one to go" when winter arrives and the colds start' (Staples, 1977).

Emotional problems do occur in boys with DMD but on the whole, they cope amazingly well. The more emotionally disturbed tend to come from families with marked conflicts and emotional problems from childhood (Staples, 1977). Emotional and/or behavioural difficulties appear to be more common in those without information about their disease or who had been told partial truths. Without a clear understanding of the existence and nature of the disease, children often blamed themselves for their 'incompetence' (Buchanan *et al.*, 1979).

Zellweger (1975) comments, 'It is worth while to emphasize that the DMD patient, after some initial frustration, is really not suffering, has above all no pain, and is on the contrary often quite content or at least acceptingly resigned after he becomes wheelchair-bound. It is the parent who suffers more than the child'.

The parents

The slow, progressive chronic illness of one family member places a demand upon all the healthy members of the family to react and adapt (Buchanan *et al.*, 1979). A family history of DMD may allow parents to anticipate the diagnosis, thereby possibly decreasing its psychological impact. Where there is no family history, one or other parent may become concerned that there is something the matter with their son. The general practitioner, finding no definite abnormality, may even consider the parents 'neurotic' and there may be considerable delay before a definitive diagnosis is made. During this time, both parents will be subject to a variable amount of anxiety brought on by the uncertainty of the situation (Firth, 1983).

The definitive diagnosis will produce a mixture of shock, denial, depression, anger and frequently relief that a diagnosis has at last been made. The expression of depression and hostility is difficult for the medical profession to cope with. Parents may appear ungrateful and unreasonable but this must be seen as a transient phase in coping.

The three coping mechanisms most frequently observed to cause problems are denial, magical thinking and over-protection. Firstly, they may refuse to believe the diagnosis (*denial*). They may seek other opinions. Some parents are unable to admit any emotional reaction whatever to DMD but can easily discuss factual material. *Magical thinking* may make parents believe that their son is different from other DMD children. They may be convinced that the condition will not progress as quickly for their son as for others or that he may even recover. *Over-protection* may be a response to a feeling of severe guilt and total helplessness. Parents may isolate the child socially, they may go to excessive lengths to buy him presents, may disregard discipline and generally infantalize him, going to extreme measures such as sleeping in the same room as their son (Buchanan *et al.*, 1979).

Coping depends, among other things, on the use the child and family have made of their disability to become a focus of other problems (Schechter, 1961). Buchanan *et al.* (1979) found 5 per cent of DMD families had marital conflict with arguments focused on caring for the child and discipline. Marital problems may be made worse by the fatigue of looking after the handicapped child, particularly the physical activity of moving the child, turning at night and coping with incontinence. As a consequence of the strain on the marriage, the couple may devote themselves to the child, never allowing themselves any break from looking after him. Others sublimate their feelings into fund raising for research and aggressively pursue the rights of handicapped people. Fathers may sometimes become detached when there is a DMD child in the family and one-third of the parents I have interviewed had great difficulty talking to each other about muscular dystrophy.

On close questioning, many parents feel that the illness was a result of some misdemeanour in their past: that they have 'sinned' (Schechter, 1961). Often, considerable guilt is felt, the parents blaming themselves for any apparent exacerbation and feeling that they are not doing enough. The most prominent psychological issue identified by parents is the unpredictability of the course of the disease. How long will the child be able to continue in school or be able to walk and when will he be bedridden (Buchanan *et al.*, 1979)? Other stresses include their son's loneliness and depression, his gradual deterioration, jealousy between normal siblings and the patient, the reaction of parents' friends and relatives towards the patient, society's attitude to handicapped people and the additional problems of mental handicap.

Siblings

Jealousy with normal siblings of the patient may cause significant distress within the family. Over-protection of the affected boy with neglect of his normal siblings is admitted by only a few parents. One survey found that 60 per cent of normal siblings experienced some degree of emotional distress. There is a tendency for older sisters to adopt a maternal role and to over-protect their affected brother while competition between brothers may pose a major problem in families where there is also a normal son (Buchanan *et al.*, 1979). Young siblings may imagine that they have magically caused any exacerbation in their brother's condition and may have to suffer some rejection by their peers.

Physical disability of later onset

There are several forms of muscular dystrophy where onset is later in adolescence or adult life and where the prognosis is better, survival often being into middle age. In these cases, the physical and concomitant psychological effects are different from DMD. The affected individual has to live and work in the community and this brings additional problems over and above those of fears of survival. A good example of such a disorder is Becker Muscular Dystrophy (BMD) which is inherited as an X-linked trait and only affects males. It is clinically somewhat similar to DMD but onset is later, usually in adolescence or early adult life, and affected males usually become confined to a wheelchair in their twenties or even thirties and survive into middle age.

Social aspects

The physical handicap is stigmatizing and affects the way in which people interact with the handicapped person. They may treat him as though intellectually impaired, speaking more loudly than usual as they might to a foreigner who has difficulty understanding the language. Frequently, their tone is patronizing. Writing about another physical condition, Sneddon (1980) commented, 'The illness caused great social embarrassment'. Many people do approach the handicapped person normally and try to treat him naturally but then become flustered when things so wrong. When holding out a hand to greet someone with muscular dystrophy, it is disconcerting to find that he is unable to extend his arm to reach your hand. In some forms of muscular dystrophy communication may be further disrupted by facial weakness: 'It is hard when people think you're miserable and you can't smile to assure them that you're not' (Sneddon, 1980).

Economic factors are undoubtedly important in the tolerance of disability (Taylor, 1978). Teenage onset and moderate severity mean that after only a few years, an affected individual will be forced to give up work with reduced income and loss of status and prestige. Within the family, his role will change from breadwinner to dependent and this change may be exacerbated if his wife starts working. Apparent demotion in family status may be evinced by children and other relatives now turning instead to his wife for advice and support.

Restricted mobility and the use of a wheelchair will limit access to some buildings for shopping, cultural and leisure purposes. Inability to afford a car will make life even more restricted and will lead the individual and his family to become socially isolated, a situation that may be heightened by friends avoiding the affected person as though he was contagious. Lack of work and mobility will leave long periods of the day to be occupied. The obvious hobbies and interests that can be pursued at home are usually impossible because of the manual dexterity required. Inevitably, there is boredom and frustration.

Perhaps the greatest social impact relates not to the lack of work or mobility, which are obvious, but to the crucial parts of daily life that most people take for granted – the ability to dress, feed, clean and generally look after oneself. Any impairment of these abilities may involve loss of privacy and modesty. Someone, usually the wife, will have to do the shopping and prepare the food, take off his night clothes and help him to dress, and will have to help him bath. When out of the house, he may be able to undo his trouser zip, but not to pull out his penis to micturate, and he may have to ask strangers to help him. He will have similar problems cleaning himself after defaecation. Ultimately, if severely handicapped and there is no relative available to look after him, he may need to be cared for in an institution.

Emotional aspects

The patient

The emotional reaction to developing a physical handicap will depend on a variety of factors including age of onset, emotional maturity, personality, nature of interpersonal relationships, intelligence, work, leisure activities and aspirations, and previous experience of handicap in the family.

In the case of BMD, the patient may appear at first to be unaware of his weakness, even though his family may hint at the problem (*denial*). He may extend himself to his physical limits as though trying to convince himself that all is well. Gradually, he will begin to admit that he is different from his peers and, if there is a family history, he may well suspect the diagnosis. This realization that something is wrong may provoke uncertainty and anxiety which may be low grade or severe and lead to panic attacks.

The maturational tasks faced by the adolescent are directed towards identity formation and his view of his identity will be closely linked to his body image. So, at a time when his peers are exploiting their growing physical prowess, he will be recognizing that his own physical strength is declining. He may consciously direct his interest to something less physical in compensation. His view of himself will colour the way he feels others must see him which in turn affects his early relationships with females. At this stage, girlfriends may be unaware of any abnormality although as time goes by, it will become apparent.

After a period of uncertainty, the diagnosis eventually will be confirmed which may bring a brief feeling of relief. The uncertainty is at an end, the doctor knows what is happening to his body and has given it a name. But his relief is usually short-lived. There is often a period of numbness and disbelief (*impact*) followed by the full reaction and social *recoil*, and eventually *reassessment* and *resolution*. The extent to which the individual successfully works through this process depends on his premorbid personality and the help and support available to him during this period.

The realization of the full meaning of the diagnosis may well be greeted with horror, revulsion, distress and a feeling of emptiness. He will grieve for his lost health, loss of prospects and hope, and the loss of a normal life. Anger is often prominent and may be directed towards all about him, especially doctors for making the diagnosis and not having a cure, and parents for having passed the condition on to him. This anger may also be directed towards himself, at the same time he is ambivalent, realizing at an intellectual level that some of these feelings are unreasonable. He may feel guilty that in some way he is responsible for the illness: 'What sin have I committed to bring this on myself?' 'I felt *unique* and *alone*. I seemed to be the only one in the world with this illness and these problems' (Carus, 1980). The married man may be convinced that his wife will leave him because of revulsion with his condition. His frame of reference has been shifted from the certainty of 'I know where I'm going as a healthy person' to an alternative uncertainty – 'I don't know what will become of me'.

As with bereavement and other normal reactions to acute stress, resolution will occur in a period of weeks or months, although some individuals will fail to adapt to the change in their lives. Mechanisms such as regression or denial, which benefit the patient in acute illness, or in the early phases of chronic illness, are generally maladaptive if the patient continues to employ them fully when the acute phase is past (Abram, 1972). Many will be left with episodes of depression and a continuing feeling of frustration and boredom.

Frustration may continue to be a major problem throughout the long course of the condition, especially in relation to being so dependent on others for every little thing. Although sexual activity may not be directly affected, loss of feeling of attractiveness may reduce sexual libido. Shoulder weakness may make masturbation impossible at a relatively early stage, heightening the feelings of frustration.

Staples (1977) studied 47 adults with muscular dystrophy and found that they tended to be more introverted than the general population but no more neurotic. Emotional problems do occur, but on the whole, patients cope with them amazingly well. The more emotionally disturbed came from families with marked conflicts and recorded disturbances from childhood.

The parents

The thought of having transmitted an abnormality to one's children often provokes feelings of guilt and anger mixed with revulsion. The way the family functions prior to the intrusion of illness is one of the most important factors determining whether shifts in relationships give rise to problems.

The wife

The couple who marry when there are few symptoms of the disease may not have anticipated the changes that will occur in their roles and relationship as the condition progresses. The marriage 'contract' – the agreed roles and responsibilities – will have to be re-negotiated and problems may arise if the wife is not prepared to accept this change. She may begin to question the marriage, wondering how she will be able to cope. She may feel let down, angry and at the same time, guilty for having these feelings which she is unable to share or explain. Unemployment may throw the couple closer together but it can also put an added strain on the relationship.

If the husband's condition is discovered after a child has been born, there will be anxiety and guilt over whether the child will be affected. Genetic counselling will inform the couple of the risks together with a variable amount of support. In the case of BMD, there is no risk of the children being affected although daughters will be carriers.,

Siblings and children

Unaffected siblings may experience 'survivor guilt' – guilt that they are normal yet their brother is affected. Frequently, siblings and other relatives may have joked about the weakness, not realizing its seriousness and implications.

Children tend not to recognize any abnormality until school age or later when they may start comparing their father with other men. At times, their questioning will be blunt and hurtful, 'Why are you not like other daddies?', 'Will I be like you when I grow up?'. They may even be resentful of the restrictions the handicap places on the family.

Counselling tasks

General considerations

The course of any chronic inherited condition can be divided into seven stages (see Table 8.1)).

It is important to assess accurately the stage reached by each family member as each may have reached a different phase of the coping process and require a different approach. It will have to be decided whether to see the family together, the parents as a couple, or the affected individual on his own.

The counsellor must be prepared to *listen*, to be sensitive to precisely what the counsellees are requesting, assess the stage they have reached in coping and the information they have received to date together with its accuracy and reality. It is important not to attempt reassurance at this stage. Members of the caring professions are trained to reduce tension, fear and unhappiness and frequently rely on their professional role to back up their reassurance. Families do not wish to be reassured: they require information and understanding. Reassurance may temporarily make them feel better but this will be short-lived and will certainly prevent the family talking about their worries in more detail.

Table 8.1   Stages of a chronic genetic condition

Stage I	Positive family history
Stage II	Abnormality notice by patient and family No diagnosis
Stage III	Abnormality confirmed by general practitioner No diagnosis
Stage IV	Diagnosis made/reaction
Stage V	Resolution/adaptation
Stage VI	Chronic handicap/progression
Stage VII	Death/grieving

The counsellor must be genuine, honest and realistic, but at the same time, leave the family with some hopes for the future. This involves talking about positives as well as negatives, achievements as well as failures. The family requires the counsellor to be able to empathize accurately, to feel that they are communicating and that someone knows what they are going through and what this experience means to them. The counsellor must, therefore, be fully conversant with the condition in all its stages, as well as the psychological and emotional effects of the disease on the affected individual and his family.

The counsellor should be consistent and able to offer some measure of continuity. Patients with chronic conditions tend to see a large number of professionals and will seldom see the same person on many occasions. Someone is required to act as co-ordinator and remain in touch with the patient and family over a long period of time.

All those involved must be alert to non-verbal communication. For example, the DMD boy who is encouraged to keep walking at home may be put in a wheelchair in hospital in order to be wheeled to the X-ray Department, giving the parents a confused message about the importance of keeping him ambulant.

In view of the acknowledged multiplicity of areas in which disturbances may arise, use of the *problem oriented approach* (Weed, 1969) is appropriate. An exhaustive list should be compiled of medical, social and psychological problems identified by the patient, his relatives as well as all the caring staff involved. In this way, both short-term plans and long-term goals can be more adequately drawn up.

Papper (1974) suggests the value of putting *plans in writing*, not only for the staff involved but also for the patient and his family. This has some value in emphasizing that, although the direct effects of the disease may be irreversible, there is a viable future for the patient and this approach may have some value in preventing problems (Taylor, 1978).

Many patients have a poor understanding of their disease because of the limited amount of information they have been given or is even available. Information may be given in writing or backed up with printed material. In any event, information must be given repeatedly although the counsellor must be sensitive to the criticism made by some families that they were given too much information too soon. Care must be taken to anticipate and correct misinformation given by relatives and friends.

One major counselling task is to encourage the frank expression of feelings. The family will need to be given the confidence that the counsellor can cope with these expressed feelings, even if they are extreme or critical. This will provide a model which the family may continue to use at home after the counselling sessions.

Specific counselling tasks (see Table 8.1)

Stage I

This is the first stage at which genetic counselling may be sought. Counsellees will be parents at risk of producing a DMD boy or, in the case of BMD, female carriers or young men at risk of developing the condition.

Counsellees must be allowed to explain why they have sought help. This is best achieved by the use of open-ended questions, except where precise factual information is required. They must be allowed to ventilate their immediate reaction to information received. The next session is an opportunity to reinforce the information and to discuss further their reactions and decisions. The experienced counsellor may be able to anticipate some of their worries. The importance of sharing their anxieties can be backed up by offering open appointments.

Stage II

At this stage, anxieties are normally kept within the family and not accessible to counselling. However, families that have previously been seen at Stage I may, at this stage, take up the option of an appointment which had previously been left open for them.

Stage III

It will usually be the family doctor who confirms that there is a significant abnormality although he may be unsure of the precise diagnosis himself. He needs to be empathic, sensitive to the patient and his family and allow all to express their reactions. He must try to balance between the reality of what he has found and leaving some hope. It might be helpful for him to explain that they may expect to experience swings from unrealistic optimism to deep despair during this period of uncertainty, and until the diagnosis is firmly established.

Stage IV

Communicating the diagnosis is of crucial importance and the management of this difficult task must be planned in advance.

In the case of DMD, both parents *must* be present and arrangements made for the affected boy to be looked after by someone else while the parents visit the clinic (Firth, 1983). It is unfair to give the parents distressing information and then expect them to leave the office and take the affected child home.

They need time before facing him. The information should be conveyed simply and at first limited to a general outline of the condition. There should be time if necessary to repeat the information. The parents must be allowed to show their immediate reaction and not be inhibited by the counsellor. Time must be allowed for recovery before leaving the clinic.

Similar arrangements are required when a diagnosis is made later in life as in BMD. The patient should be invited to come with a close relative or with his wife if he is married.

At the end of the session, a follow-up meeting should be arranged. It may be helpful to give counsellees permission to telephone if they wish prior to the next meeting.

At the second meeting, open-ended questions are used to assess the emotional reaction to diagnosis and the amount of information retained. In response to questioning, more information can be given. They should be invited to verbalize their feelings, including those that are negative or critical. It should be made clear that this is a normal, healthy reaction to distressing circumstances and they should be encouraged not to seek medication to 'treat' their distress. Additional support may be useful although not necessarily welcome at this stage. 'We didn't particularly want this help at this time, but it came to us and we benefitted from it a lot. Probably at that particular time, people are more in need of help than at any other. If we had gone through that period, we could have resisted contact with others. I think in the first few days or couple of weeks when you find out, are the times when people can be helped most'.

Stage V

During the phase of resolution and adaptation to altered circumstances, continuity of care is important. Distressing conditions are frequently delegated to others for continued care. This is not in the best interests of the patient or family. Sessions should set the model of open communication which can be continued at home. Planning is goal-oriented and the counsellor will have to assess which long-term goals can be tackled. In the case of DMD, it appears that fathers more frequently wish to make detailed plans for their son's future.

A system of professional and voluntary support may be offered but the counsellor should be sensitive to the informal support system that the patient's family already has. Professional support can sometimes be seen to devalue and undermine the local informal support already available. The question of independence is important if over-protection is to be avoided. Parents must be encouraged to take time off from looking after their handicapped youngster and have a regular time set aside for themselves. They must learn to focus on the positives and the present. They should not dwell on the past or past achievements and their fantasies about the future need to be talked about and tempered with reality.

The physically handicapped child must be allowed to talk about his frustrations, disappointments, depression and anxieties for the future. Many people, including parents, do not allow the child to talk about these areas for fear of putting ideas into his head. The ideas certainly are there already but most children are denied the opportunity of communicating them to others. This may make them feel more isolated and abnormal because it prevents others from empathizing accurately with their position. Groups of similarly affected adolescents may allow a freer sharing of ideas and worries and a range of topics which most people are frightened of raising can be discussed, such as sexual frustration, masturbation and thoughts about death.

The adult with physical handicap needs to be seen in his own right as well as with his wife. There are certain things he has to work out as an individual and others which can only be tackled in the context of his marriage. In all events, counselling and emotional support cannot be divorced from offers of practical help. Out-patient clinics tend to focus on the 'patient' and ignore relatives. The wife will need support in her own right in these sessions and must be encouraged to have time to herself away from her caring role.

Stage VI

As the DMD boy becomes physically more debilitated in his late teens, the family must be prepared for death which may occur suddenly as a result of any minor infection. Much grief work can be done in anticipation during this stage. Again, it is a matter of encouraging the family to look at what is happening and to talk honestly about their emotional reactions: their distress, anger, despair, as well as such feelings as the wish that it was all over and that the boy was no longer suffering. During this stage, if the boy remains at home, he will require a considerable amount of physical help, such as turning at night. A great deal of general support will also be needed. The child, the adolescent or adult who is declining often turns in on himself, becoming depressed, uncommunicative and withdrawn. Parents and wives frequently 'look on the bright side', distracting the individual as much as possible from his plight and are frightened to ask what he is feeling for fear of showing their own distress. These boys and men have the right to talk about what is happening to them and their fears, if they choose to do so. They should be given opportunities to talk but it is not helpful to force the issue. It is important to make sure that these opportunities to talk about decline and death are real and that the verbal cues are not negated by the non-verbal message that this is something not to be talked about. Counselling does not end with the death of the patient but should be available to close relatives until the grieving has passed.

General conclusions

I have recently completd a survey of DMD families in the Edinburgh region and the co-operation of the parents in these families was most impressive. Some commented that this was the first time they had systematically talked about the child's problems in such detail and their own way of coping. Some said that it was to be the start of a continuing process. The investigation and the interest appeared to have therapeutic significance for these parents. In line with Barsch (1968), I consider that the general tendency to characterize parents of handicapped children as guilt-ridden, anxiety-laden, over-protective and rejecting beings is unfortunate. While it is true that such cases exist, the majority of parents are unduly stigmatized by this generalization. This type of notion calls for a preconceived approach to a therapeutic relationship which almost defies the patient to accept the generalization (Barsch, 1968). It is possible to have a handicapped child without rejecting him or becoming over-protective or guilt-ridden. Most parents in my study had outside social interests and where this was not true of a particular parent, the evidence did not suggest that the limitation of social activity held a significant relationship to the fact that the family contained a handicapped child.

References

Abram, H. S. (1972). The Psychology of Chronic Illness. *J. Chronic Diseases* **25**, 659–664.

Barsch, R. H. (1968). 'The Parent of the Handicapped Child'. Charles C. Thomas, Springfield, Illinois.

Bayrakal, S. (1975). A Group Experience with Chronically Disabled Adolescents. *Am. J. Psychiat.* **132**, 1291–1294.

Bossingham, D. H.., Williams, E., Nichols, P. J. R. (1977). 'Severe Childhood Neuromuscular Disease'. Muscular Dystrophy Group of Great Britain, London.

Buchanan, D. C., Labarbera, C. J., Roelofs, R., Olson, W. (1979). Reactions of Families to Children with Duchenne Muscular Dystrophy. *Gen. Hosp. Psychiat.* **1**, 262–269.

Carus, R. (1980). Motor Neurone Disease: A Demeaning Illness. *Br. Med. J.* **280**, 455–456.

Emery, A. E. H. (1980). Duchenne Muscular Dystrophy: Genetic Aspects. *Br. Med. Bull.* **36**, 117–122.

Firth, M. A. (1983). Diagnosis of Duchenne Muscular Dystrophy: experiences of parents of sufferers. *Br. Med. J.* **286**, 700–701.

Fischman, S. E. (1979). Psychological Issues in Genetic counselling of Cystic Fibrosis. *In* 'Genetic Counselling, Psychological Dimension' (S. Kessler, Ed.), pp. 153–166. Academic Press, New York.

Gardner-Medwin, D. (1975). The Effects of Genetic Counselling in Duchenne Muscular Dystrophy. *In* 'Recent Advances in Myology – Proceedings of the Third International Congress on Muscle Diseases' (W. G. Bradley, D. Gardner-Medwin and J. N. Walton, Eds), pp. 471–478. Excerpta Medica, Amsterdam.

Goffman, E. (1963). 'Stigma: Notes on the Management of a Spoiled Identity'. Prentice-Hall, New York (reprinted 1968, Penguin Books, London, pp. 1–40).

Morgan, G. (1975). The Effects of Genetic Counselling in Duchenne Muscular Dystrophy. *In* 'Recent Advances in Myology – Proceedings of the Third International Congress on Muscle Diseases' (W. G. Bradley, D. Gardner-Medwin and J. N. Walton, Eds), pp. 471–478. Excerpta Medica, Amsterdam.

Nichols, P. J. R. (1971). Some problems in rehabilitation of the severely disabled. *Proc. R. Soc. Med.* **64**, 349–353.

Papper, S. (1974). A 'Program' for the Chronically Ill. *J. Chronic Diseases* **27**, 175–176.

Schechter, M. D. (1961). The Orthopaedically Handicapped Child: Emotional Reactions. *Arch. Gen. Psychiat.* **4**, 247–253.

Sneddon, J. (1980). Myasthenia Gravis: A Study of Social, Medical and Emotional Problems in Twenty-six Patients. *Lancet* **1**, 526–528.

Staples, D. (1977). Intellect and Psychological Problems. *In* 'Severe Childhood Neuromuscular Disease' (D. H. Bossingham, E. Williams and P. J. R. Nichols, Eds), pp. 30–32. Muscular Dystrophy Group of Great Britain, London.

Taylor, P. C. (1978). Psychological Disturbance in Adults with Chronic Physical Illness. *In* 'Current Themes in Psychiatry' (R. Gaind and B. Hudson, Eds), pp. 180–189. Macmillan Press, London.

Vignos, P. J. (1975). The Comprehensive Management of Duchenne Muscular Dystrophy. *In* 'Recent Advances in Mycology – Proceedings of the Third International Congress on Muscle Diseases' (W. G. Bradley, D. Gardner-Medwin and J. N. Walton, Eds), pp. 455–461. Excerpta Medica, Amsterdam.

Weed, L. L. (1969). Medical Records, Medical Education and Patient Care. Press of Case Western Reserve University, Cleveland.

Wyngaarden, J. B. and Smith, L. H. (1982). 'Cecil: Textbook of Medicine'. W. B. Saunders, Philadelphia.

Zellweger, H. (1975). Family Counselling in Duchenne Muscular Dystrophy. *In* 'Recent Advances in Myology – Proceedings of the Third International Congress on Muscle Diseases' (W. G. Bradley, D. Gardner-Medwin and J. N. Watson, Eds), pp. 469–471. Excerpta Medica, Amsterdam.

9 Huntington's Disease and Other Late Onset Genetic Disorders

NANCY S. WEXLER

I am not resigned to the shutting away of loving hearts in the hard ground.
So it is, and so it will be, for so it has been, time out of mind:
Into the darkness they go, the wise and the lovely. Crowned
With lilies and with laurel they go; but I am not resigned.

Edna St. Vincent Millay: Dirge Without Music

Introduction

In a laboratory at Rockefeller University, New York, research is underway on the psychophysiology of stress. Three rats are confined side by side in nearly identical narrow boxes, a turning wheel in front of them and electrodes attached to their tails. The first two animals are 'yoked' together so that their tail electrodes lead to a common source and fire together. The control animal's tail electrode is not attached to an electrical stimulus. All three animals hear a signal. The 'avoidance-escape' rat moves quickly to turn his wheel and avoid a shock. If he is too slow, both he and his 'yoked' partner receive identical shocks. At the end of the experiment, the control animal has virtually no gastric lesions while the avoidance-escape animal has some. The 'helpless' yoked animal, however, who receives exactly the same number of shocks as his partner but is totally unable to control his situation, has almost four times as many severe gastric lesions. In addition, the yoked animal subjected to uncontrollable shocks gradually stops eating and drinking, loses weight, becomes lethargic and performs poorly on active motor tasks, becomes passive and non-competitive, ceases grooming and play activity, sleeps less – in short, looks as close as an animal can to being depressed (Weiss, 1977, 1980, 1982).

Imagine, if you will, this experiment in nature. Instead of rats in separate compartments, imagine a family 'yoked' together invisibly by their common genetic background. What happens to one affects unpredictably and uncontrollably one or more of the others. The shock may or may not come, and for some, the experiment isn't fully over until life itself is finished.

The investigations of Jay M. Weiss and colleagues at Rockefeller University and others in stress research would predict that many 'at risk' for inheriting a late onset genetic disorder are in situations which produce maximal stress: unpredictably, lack of control, and prolonged confinement in the stressful condition with no means of escape.

Huntington's disease

Huntington's disease provides a classic example. As an autosomal dominant late onset disorder, each child of a parent with Huntington's disease has a 50 per cent chance of inheriting the condition. But there is no test that can detect the presence of the gene until symptoms of the disease appear. The usual age of onset is in the third or fourth decade, but the disease may make its insidious debut even in childhood or remain quiescent until the 80s. This means that parents begin to watch their children at a very young age and continue to do so until the disease, their child's death, or their own death intervenes. It is difficult to be totally confident that the illness has disappeared unless autopsies are performed on those at risk and several gene-free generations have passed. The gene is fully penetrant and never skips a generation. Huntington's disease eventually is terminal after ten to twenty years of progressive disability. There is no effective treatment. Individuals watch themselves, watch their sibs, watch their parents, watch their children.

Huntington's disease has a tripartite symptomatology which affects almost every aspect of functioning – the three M's: movement, mood and mentation. The body gradually becomes engulfed in a panoply of abnormal movements – chorea, dystonia, rigidity, tremor, athetosis, tics, grimaces – until voluntary movement is superceded by constant, involuntary motion. Mood is altered, usually becoming depressed sometimes to the point of suicide, occasionally becoming manic, often irritable, explosive, hypersensitive, withdrawn and apathetic. Auditory or visual hallucinations may occur. Thinking, reasoning, organizing and planning become disrupted, judgement goes awry, memory is impaired but some insight into their own and family members' conditions and even a sense of humor can be maintained until the end. Speech is lost, independent care is impossible, choking is frequent and death may be a welcome relief (Wexler, 1979).

Huntington's disease may be a particularly dramatic model of the problems associated with late onset disorders, but it by no means has a monopoly on these difficulties. Patients with dominantly inherited olivopontocerebellar atrophy (OPCA) or recessively transmitted Friedreich's and other ataxias often have married and produced a family before the tell-tale signs of cerebellar incoordination begin to appear and the next generation starts its vigil. Joseph's disease patients and others with similar spinocerebellar degenerations develop, in their twenties and thirties, a wide-based gait, incoordination, and slow progression to total incapacity and death. The child over 12 at risk for dominant polyposis is screened each year for the sinister polyps which herald the onset of colon malignancy but which can save lives if caught soon enough as harbingers of the gene (McKusick, 1976).

As understanding of genetics has grown, many more illnesses are recognized as having a genetic component. Amyotrophic lateral sclerosis (ALS or Lou Gerhig's disease) is a mid-life degenerative disorder of motor neurons producing progressive muscle weakness and paralysis. After a period of two to ten years the patient dies, usually of respiratory failure. A rare hereditary variant of ALS appears as an autosomal dominant disorder with late onset (McKusick, 1976). Schizophrenia in a parent increases the child's risk for the disorder from the 1 to 2 per cent for the general population to 12 to 14 per cent or even 35 to 45 per cent if both parents are unlucky enough to manifest the illness (Garmezy, 1980). Typically, schizophrenia emerges in the late teens, although onset is slightly older for girls. Manic-depressive disorder also has a strong genetic component (Garmezy, 1980). The heart attack victim below the age of 40 may have autosomal dominant, late onset familial hypercholesterolemia (McKusick, 1976). Others discover, to their horror, that their fragile, elderly relative in the nursing home has Alzheimer's disease (a form of senile dementia) and may have a 50 per cent probability of passing on this terrifying illness. Although perhaps the majority of cases of Alzheimer's disease are sporadic, as people are living longer and inheritance patterns can be seen more clearly, it is evident that in some families this classically late onset disorder is transmitted as an autosomal dominant (Heston, Bar Harbor Alzheimer's Disease Conference, in press).

> The beginning of an acquaintance whether with persons or things is to get a definite outline for our ignorance.
>
> George Eliot (Mary Ann Evans): Daniel Deronda

The genetic counselor (or whatever medical professional is responsible for providing genetic counseling) has the complex task of explaining the genetic nature of these conditions to those affected by them, either actually or potentially. I would like to make a radical proposal to these counselors: devote yourselves wholeheartedly to prevention. The role of the genetic counselor has changed appreciably in recent history. In the days of Davenport and the Social Darwinists, genetic counseling was the simple purveying of genetic facts, usually with a eugenic aim. As World War II and the apex of eugenic zeal passed, eugenics lost favor and 'psychological mindedness', honed by coping with the traumas of war, took its place. The role of genetic counseling was broadened to include in its scope the need to help individuals and couples assimilate and adjust to the information they learned, particularly with a view toward helping them make better informed reproductive decisions (Wexler, 1980). But does this new definition of genetic counseling go far enough? Or are we diagnosing an illness and leaving the patient untreated?

I do not mean to imply a return to Social Darwinism and eugenics when I advocate prevention. Rather, I urge that counselors pursue an active plan to prevent the traumatic psychological and even physical sequelae that almost inevitably follow a diagnosis of serious genetic disease. One can predict – almost guarantee – that the discovery of certain conditions in families will produce severe distress and emotional turmoil. Yet, counselors assume that most families can handle the strain or will seek help if they cannot. Why do we take these things for granted? Why do we assume that people know how to cope without being taught? Why do we force individuals to request to come to us for further help when to do so often is experienced by them as an admission of failure to cope independently? The British hospice movement should teach us a lesson about preventive interventions. When dying cancer patients in a hospice were given pain medication prophylactically, on a regular schedule, patients could relax and not dread the onset of pain. There was no internal struggle about when to request pain medication, when to admit it was getting bad, no apprehension that the pain would mount to intolerable levels before relief was administered. As a result, patients felt psychologically secure and their consumption of the prophylactic analgesic decreased.

If a person is diagnosed as having a serious medical illness, follow-up care with a physician is usually required and the doctor has some opportunity to observe how the person is coping. But in a genetic disease, a client may come for genetic counseling, receive the appropriate information and never be heard from again. Who knows if the information was assimilated, comprehended, or managed emotionally? There are innumerable stories of families traumatized by genetic information. Many suffer needlessly from misinformation and misconceptions while others flounder with a novel psychological situation which they are ill prepared to understand or handle. The divorce rate among couples struggling with genetic illness exceeds the national average and tales abound in the literature of psychological casualties (Leonard et al., 1972).

Genetic counselors are in a perfect position to observe how people cope successfully and unsuccessfully with genetic information and to teach their clients the best methods. Counselors should develop an active program of outreach and prevention.

In our current practice, a couple may or may not return for additional sessions with a counselor once a diagnosis is made. If the couple is undergoing amniocentesis or has just suffered the birth of an infant with a genetic disorder, they may be supported temporarily by a net of medical personnel handling the medical situation. But for others, the genetic facts may be communicated quickly, after which the client disappears from view. Children at risk for OPCA or Joseph's disease or Huntington's disease may have only one or two sessions with a counselor. If not referred to a neurologist for follow-up care, they may never discuss the illness with a knowledgeable person able to correct misconceptions or help them adjust to the psychological burden.

Many at risk for late onset diseases only receive counseling from their parents, who may be poorly informed or ill equipped to help the child cope. Voluntary health agencies are extremely valuable in providing support and some have family discussion groups, but relying on other organizations to provide needed services given by well trained service providers is haphazard at best.

The genetic counseling field can learn from the experience of Chinese psychiatry. Chinese psychiatrists were appalled at the 30–40 per cent readmission rate of their patients following two to three months of psychiatric hospitalization. They instituted a vigorous follow-up program and insisted that patients return with their families to the hospital as outpatients for follow-up care once a month for the first year following hospitalization, and every two months for the second year. Letters of reminder were sent to the patient before each visit, and if the patient failed to return, a hospital worker went on a home visit. The relapse rate dropped dramatically to 10–16 per cent (Personal Communication: Dr Wu Chen-i, Director of An Ding Hospital, Beijing).

I certainly do not mean to imply that all families with a genetic disorder will become mentally ill. But a genetic counselor usually only sees the family at the crisis moment of diagnosis. The counselor has no way of knowing how families adjust after several months or even several years, when children are in different stages of the life cycle and have changed pressures as well as resources.

In Wales, geneticist Peter Harper, working closely with a social worker, has an active outreach program with a large number of Huntington's disease families. They see all families in the area once every year. Much to their surprise, they discovered that the birth rate among those at risk declined markedly. Regular opportunities to discuss the illness and the availability of knowledgeable people for crisis intervention seemed to ease psychological tensions and allow couples to abide by decisions not to procreate that they had made on their own, not from any directive of the counselors (Harper *et al.*, 1979).

The norm for genetic counseling should be multiple sessions at the time of initial counseling, not only to take a proper pedigree and make the correct diagnosis, but also to educate fully monitoring the retention of information, and to discuss psychological responses. Many centers currently follow this practice. Additionally, follow-up sessions should be scheduled semi-annually or annually, like an annual physical or Pap (cervical smear) test. Obviously, if the client has a good relationship with another physician or counselor who serves the same function, these visits are unnecessary. For purposes of discussion, I am disregarding problems of financial reimbursement or personnel which can make the best of intentions impossible to realize. Rather, I would like to stress a change in attitude toward the counseling, an attitude which emphasizes that psychological reactions are the norm and should be anticipated, that dealing with them takes time and that genetic counselors have an obligation to assist clients with these reactions and should acquire the training and information necessary.

> O gentlemen, the time of life is short;
> To spend that shortness basely were too long
> If life did ride upon a dial's point,
> Still ending at the arrival of an hour.
>
> *Shakespeare: Henry IV*

There is a large literature on stress and its management that is useful for counselors to learn and to teach to their clients. Genetic counselors are familiar with stressful elements unique to the genetic situation which should enable them to help their clients anticipate and manage these pressures more effectively. Extrapolating from research findings on stress, the following are some suggestions for ways in which counselors can help their clients accommodate to their genetic situation.

Make explicit the psychology of the illness

The genetic counselor should be familiar with the psychological reactions triggered by specific genetic illnesses. Some are common to many people affected by the disorder, some are unique to particular individuals and stem from their idiosyncratic histories. Counselors should listen for the client's interpretation of the illness. Usually it is beneficial to make the client's perceptions explicit, particularly if they are incorrect, and reflect aloud on the meaning the illness seems to hold for the client. Many people have a well defended, rational image of the disorder and, simultaneously, a collage of partially formed images, reemergences of hidden fears, secret meanings of a dire and ominous sort, reverberations with past traumas. It may also be helpful for clients to know that they are not alone in their reactions, both accurate and inaccurate.

Each aspect of the illness in question is involved in determining the psychological impact of the disorder and should be considered.

Variation in age of onset and the development of symptoms

The age of onset of a disease will radically affect emotional reactions to it. If the disease starts at a young age, the counselor mainly works with healthy parents or sibs dealing with their concern for a sick or potentially ill child. The counselor typically does not work with the individual destined for the genetic illness. If the illness has a later age of onset, the picture is more complex. The counselor may see as clients multiple generations at once, the parents, children – grown up and young – and spouses of older offspring. The counselor may be speaking to someone who either has or potentially has passed on a gene or to the actual or potential recipient of the gene. The client may be healthy, may be affected, may be in limbo between both states with an unclear diagnosis.

Many feelings are shared by 'early onset' families and 'late onset' families. Parents in both feel guilty about passing on a damaging or even lethal gene to their offspring, even if there is no objective basis for their guilt. Many experience the appearance of genetic disease as a punishment for transgressions, often sexual – an affair, an abortion – or as some indication that they are defective.

The major difference between early and late onset families is the extraordinary prolongation of an ambiguous and stressful situation in the latter. Huntington's disease is a graphic case in point. For many, the delayed age of onset allows them to rejoice in the healthy years of their children, parents, or themselves. For others, however, there is a lingering suspicion that the gene may really begin its work at birth but be undetectable until later, except to the very wary, watchful eye. A delayed age of onset with no early diagnostic test and insidious first symptoms produces a family in chronic stress. Counselors can teach some specific ways in which at-risk individuals and other family members can manage this stress:

Recognize normal behavior

Counselors should teach clients how to discriminate between normal behavior and abnormal behavior. The normal range of clumsiness, mood swings, memory lapses, or other possible symptoms of Huntington's disease and a variety of other late onset diseases is generally much greater than most realize. When individuals suddenly discover they are at risk, they often become hyper-alert to normal behavior which they never had occasion to notice in themselves. The counselor can teach about myoclonic jerks, and warn that they will no doubt begin to notice when they walk into walls, stumble, forget phone numbers, or do a variety of other normal behaviors.

Learn baseline functioning

Teach individuals to know their own baselines. Different people vary widely in their grace, coordination, intellectual talent, etc. The most important aspect for recognizing a late onset disorder is a *change*, a *progressive deterioration*, in normal baseline functioning. Everyone has normal fluctuations and lapses but the hallmark of illness is a steady decline. If there is no progressive change, the likelihood is that nothing is wrong.

Avoid 'symptom seeking'

Discuss 'symptom seeking' and try to ease the pressure on individuals who become hypervigilant in looking for early signs. If the disease arrives, they will know soon enough. For many people at risk, the illness is often in the back of their minds. A new challenge, physical or intellectual, also can be seen as a test of their state of health. Learning to play tennis, skiing for the first time, balancing on a log while hiking or learning to use a computer can be a test to determine if the gene is there and at work. The exhilaration of conquering a new skill is magnified by this secret test, but so too is the pressure on the novice. A counselor can be of assistance by tactfully discussing with at-risk individuals the private hoops they create for themselves to jump through and thereby may ease the tension of being chronically tested.

Attend to general health

Improve health in general. Although there is no indication that good general health can stave off the illness or make it any less severe, neither is there research in this area. Common sense would dictate that good physical and mental health would stand anyone with a chronic condition in good stead. Excessive alcohol is deleterious to the body and particularly the brain, and seems to exacerbate the symptoms of some diseases, such as Huntington's disease. Good nutrition, normal weight, no smoking, and exercise should all be maintained. Those who become ill, as well as those who do not, will benefit by adhering to these guidelines. Furthermore, the active maintenance of good health is something which individuals themselves can undertake to gain some sense of mastery and control over their lives in addition to benefiting their health.

Transmission pattern

The transmission pattern of an illness is a major aspect of its psychology. If a disease is recessive, both parents 'share the blame' equally. Both parents have identical responsibility, although couples have been known to deny this fact. An X-linked disease imposes a particular strain on an asymptomatic female carrier of the illness. The carrier does not need to fear getting the disorder herself, but she bears the full genetic burden of passing on a defective gene. Even if a carrier mother and normal father both decide to risk having children, it is the mother who knows that a son with hemophilia or muscular dystrophy suffers because of something in her genome. This can cause great strain on a marriage and family ties. Carrier sisters of an affected boy have, in addition to normal sibling rivalry, the knowledge of invulnerability that their additional X chromosome provides; but they also know that they have the power to inflict the same fate on a son of theirs that they witness in a loved brother.

An autosomal dominant illness lays the onus of guilt again on the shoulders of just one parent. Unless the disorder is produced by a new mutation, the affected offspring shares the disease with the affected parent. This can increase the identification of the child with that parent – for better or worse – and also permit the child to observe the illness in someone else. Problems may arise if the offspring is more severely affected than the parent, for example, if the parent has only a few 'café au lait' spots and the child has severe neurofibromatosis. If the illness has fairly early onset, the child can observe how the affected parent copes with the disorder and learn firsthand that it is possible to make one's way in the world, to fall in love, get married and have children with such a condition.

If the disorder has delayed onset, the relationship between parent and child is quite different. The still normal child witnesses in the parent what he or she may become. If there is an early diagnostic test, the child knows the fate to expect. If there is no such test, as is more often the case, the child is torn between identifying with a sick parent in whose footsteps he or she might follow or denying the ill parent and any similarity which might suggest that the child shares a genetic bond.

The child lives in a situation in which the affected parent is like a living mirror of the child's own future. Children often feel enraged with a parent who placed them in 'genetic jeopardy' and at the same time are deeply sympathetic and distraught over the plight of a loved and dying parent, particularly one whom they knew in healthier years. Unfortunately, most delayed onset disorders are autosomal dominant.

Symptomatology

The most crucial aspect of understanding the psychology of the disease is to appreciate the nature of the threat posed by its symptoms. What is lost by having this disease? What does the illness attack? There will be both universal and personal reactions to different types of symptoms. For example, those at risk for autosomal dominant polyposis know that there is a 50 per cent probability that cells within their colon will turn cancerous. The disease can be caught early when only polyps are forming and prophylactic treatment by colectomy is quite effective, but the cancer scare is real and the colectomy must be done at an early age, with all the attendant problems this can cause for children and young adults. Breast cancer in women can be strongly hereditary in certain families, imposing the difficult psychological choice of prophylactic double mastectomies on some young women who are still dating, unmarried and childless. Families at risk for familial hypercholesterolemia live under the constant threat of sudden, lethal heart attack. Retinitis pigmentosa gene carriers have a future of blindness to dread.

To those at risk for, or in the early stages of, Huntington's disease, the attack is on all fronts. Understandably, the suicide rate in these patients is seven times the national average (Commission for the Control of Huntington's Disease and Its Consequences, 1977). Huntington's disease symptomatology attacks the essence of what makes us human. One woman learned in her early thirties that she was at risk for Huntington's disease. She managed tolerably well with this information until her mother began showing signs of paranoia and serious mental illness. Then she panicked. As long as she felt that she could rely on a competent mind to cope with the illness, she could tolerate it. But to see her mother's mind 'go' and fear that the same would happen to her was terrifying. When she could discuss her worst fears about the disease with an expert and empathic neurologist who explained to her the variability in symptomatology and took *time* to listen sympathetically, her fears subsided.

In an analogous example, a man at risk had his rigidly held defenses against the disease shattered as an adolescent when he watched aghast as his once beautiful mother stood at the kitchen sink attempting to wash dishes while urine rolled down her leg and on to the floor.

There is a very large Huntington's disease kindred in Venezuela who describe their disorder in a special way. They say that every offspring of an

Huntington's disease parent has inherited the disorder but that only certain individuals will get sick. This distortion of genetic fact accurately expresses an emotional truth: those at risk for Huntington's disease have inherited some constant potential to manifest the disease and in that sense are not entirely normal, but they may or may not become ill depending on various circumstances. To inherit Huntington's disease is for the Venezuelans a separate and unique state apart from having Huntington's disease. At-risk individuals inherit it; affected individuals have it.

A family disorder: 'Six Characters in Search of an Author'

The one certain aspect of a genetic disease is that it is a family disorder. There are many players in the family drama, all with their own point of view, their own threat, their own fears, their own capabilities. Like the lost and lonely characters of Pirandello's play, each actor searches for an author to write a central unifying theme and give expression to his or her particular point of view. In recessive disorders the cast can be fairly small. But in dominant disorders, particularly those of late onset, there can be a cast of hundreds.

The genetic counselor does not necessarily have the crucial cast of characters in the office. It may be wise to ask as many as is practical to come in so that each can have a better appreciation of the entire family dynamics. There are the critical and blaming parents and in-laws, the parents who feel guilty, whether healthy or affected, siblings who are convinced that some one of them must have the gene – like the proverbial hot potato – but who don't want it to be themselves and feel guilty about 'giving' it to a sib. There are cousins on the affected side who share the same concerns and cousins on the unaffected side who are envied and are, perhaps, a little more distant. There are always 'watchers' in late onset disorder families, the hypervigilant who don't want any surprises, who mask their dismay and horror at seeing the disease appear by smug, self-satisfaction at recognizing it first.

Some families tacitly elect a delegate to represent them at the genetic counselor's sessions. Some have the official 'copers' and the official black sheep who won't visit an affected parent, won't go to voluntary health organization meetings, see doctors or talk about the illness. Each family has its own Florence Nightingale and its own Cain and Abel. The genetic counselor must try to see the disease from the point of view of each of these characters, whether they are present in the office or merely described, and observe how their attitudes affect the entire family's adjustment to the genetic situation. The counselor may have to translate for other family members to enable them to empathize with relatives whose points of view may be unclear. In a family disease, all members of the family have a story but sometimes each is involved in delivering a soliloquy. The counselor may have to write the script.

> To have in general but little feeling, seems to be the only security against feeling too much on any particular occasion.
>
> *George Eliot (Mary Ann Evans): Middlemarch*

The 'doyen' of stress research, Dr Hans Selye, describes a field of 'stress-ology' but claims that although everyone talks about it, no one defines it. His own definition is 'the *nonspecific* that is, common *result of any demand upon the body*, be the effect mental or somatic' (Selye, 1982). Selye's stressors are an array of noxious, positive or neutral events which tax the body's resources. Other investigators have included the notion of overload: 'stress occurs in the face of demands that tax or exceed the resources of the system or . . . to which there are no readily available or automatic adaptive responses' (Selye, 1982).

Two interrelated stresses which appear to be universally taxing from the first stages of development are lack of control and the fear of being over-whelmed. Both these stresses and others are frequent in families 'hosting' late onset genetic disorders. Feeling helpless can lead to hopelessness and depres-sion, both in experimental animals and in man, which can in turn make the organism more vulnerable to disease and prolong recovery from disorders contracted. The fear of being flooded and overwhelmed by uncontrollable feelings, of being engulfed by painful and unmanageable emotions of rage or despair or grief often leads people to put a very tight rein on feelings which fester under wraps. These feelings may break out at inappropriate times, with inappropriate people, or lead to intrusive, obsessional thoughts, nightmares, phobias, headaches or other psychosomatic complaints. In certain families, early screening for cancer or heart disease gives an individual a means of actively interceding in the disease. But other families have absolutely no control over the appearance of the illness. For Huntington's disease families, this lack of control is experienced as one of the most diabolical features of the illness.

For some individuals, the stress of ambiguity is worse than the life threatening aspect of the disease itself. In an attempt to manage this ambiguity and the totally random nature of genetic transmission, people often concoct private explanations which give the situation some order in their own minds, even if they pay a tremendous cost for their psychological resolution.

A colleague of mine described how at the age of 12 he had been playing a vigorous game of baseball with his father after which his father collapsed and died of a heart attack. Since all the males in his family on his father's side had similarly died before the age of 42, my colleague assumed his fate would be the same. Intellectually he knew that some 'bad gene' was segregating in his family, although he didn't know its name was familial hypercholesterolemia.

He had never gone for genetic counseling or even for a medical check-up, in part because emotionally he felt responsible for precipitating his father's death, even though rationally he understood that he was in no way to blame.

He determined to make a mark for himself early in life and before the age of 40 became the chairman of a prestigious university department. Despite this intellectual achievement, he had never been able to mourn the loss of his father since to do so overwhelmed him with guilt and longing and dread over his own future. Every time he thought of the future, he panicked at the thought of sudden death. The only way he could endure the terror of the waiting game was to take matters actively into his own hands to ensure that he would control the outcome: he became massively obese. He would 'get it' before 'it got him'.

Finally, with the help of a therapist whose secure relationship made it safer to face the abyss of his future, he realized he was committing suicide rather than face uncertainty. He began to opt for life. He hadn't killed his father, he didn't need to expiate his father's death with his own, he could permit himself to crave life instead of stifling these hopeless longings with food. He might even have some control over his future if he was willing to take a risk. He lost 100 pounds, began to exercise. Days after his 39th birthday he died of a massive coronary. Someone should have gotten to him sooner.

> My desolation does begin to make
> A better life.
> *Shakespeare: Antony and Cleopatra*

Counselors can become infected by their clients' sense of despair and futility if they are not adequately trained to protect themselves as well as the client. At a genetic counseling course a young student confessed that she 'dreaded working with Huntington's disease families because there is nothing that can be done'. Another counselor spoke of working with a man suffering from another hereditary progressive neurological disease who complained that he kept waiting 'for the other shoe to fall' and the disease to get worse. So did the counselor. Both these two young counselors were falling into the same fallacies as their clients – that the only thing to do was to make the disease go away. For the counselors and clients, everything was perceived in terms of the disease so that everything was seen as hopeless.

The counselor's main goal in helping clients deal with the stress of late onset genetic disease is to help give them a sense of control over their lives, even if they cannot control the gene, and to reduce the feeling of being overwhelmed.

One effective way of doing this is to teach clients to be flexible and to redefine their goals. If a vision of a crushing future of dying parents, compromised marriage, repudiated children, economic insecurity and career doubt leads to paralysis and depression, help the person set smaller, daily goals which can be mastered with pride. Teach how to live one day at a time without being oblivious to certain concerns for the future such as medical insurance, contraception, economic planning and other specific activities. It is not sufficient merely to tell someone to live step by step – one must instruct the person in how to set realistic goals, work toward accomplishing them, and, most importantly, shift set if need be. In an impossible situation, sometimes the best goal is to develop a sense of humor.

> Life is not a matter of holding good cards, but of playing a poor hand well.
> *Robert Louis Stevenson*

An indirect way to help people modify their own behavior is to teach them how to help someone else do the same. Entire families are often disrupted by the frustration and despair of the handicapped patient who no longer can do previously easy chores. For example, one 28 year old mother with Huntington's disease attempted suicide in part because she could no longer clean the house as before and felt useless and depressed. A counselor worked with the mother and her 10 year old daughter to set a weekly schedule for cleaning – one thing each day, no less and also no more. The daughter colored a bright calendar of duties for them both, posted it on the refrigerator where it could not be missed and each applied gold stars for tasks accomplished. In this very concrete way, the mother's goals were subdivided into structured units of time – her ultimate goal still being to clean the house – the daughter also learned how to set smaller, realistic goals, and both had a good time inventing a kind of game which brought them closer together.

Teaching clients a new perspective on time can be particularly valuable in helping them cope with reproductive decisions. If couples perceive a yawning future full of aching and barren years stretching before them, a natural instinct is to populate those years as rapidly as possible. How much easier it is to wait one year and see how research progresses. Particularly if couples are young and can afford to take their time, they will find it far more comfortable to give up procreation for a year with the hope of change than to think of forsaking reproduction for the rest of their lives. After several years, some marriages dissolve, some couples adopt if they are able, and others find that their desire for children has diminished. There are still a surprising number of medical personnel who advise people at risk for Huntington's disease to get sterilized immediately and not even to contemplate having children. A far better effect may be achieved by breaking the future into smaller 'pieces' and encouraging couples to refrain for a year, see how they feel, and then come back again to discuss it.

The investigators developed 'a profound sense of awe at the biological tough-
ness of the human spirit.'

A. Roe and B. Burks

Genetic counseling as a discipline is relatively young. The conceptualiza-
tion of genetic counseling as the provision of prophylactic preventive intervention is newer yet. There are some scientists, however, who have thought
diligently about the problems of high risk families, families in slums, poverty
families, immigrant families, above all, children of parents with serious
psychiatric disease. These children are compromised by a possible genetic
load, experience disrupted parenting from a highly disturbed individual and
often live in poor social and economic circumstances because the affected
parent may be the bread winner or cost a great deal in medical bills, or be
generally socially disruptive. In studying children from these malignant
backgrounds, investigators became curious about the children who survived
or even transcended their environment relatively unscathed. Instead of
offering tepid sympathy to disadvantaged children, they set about to learn the
ingredients of 'invulnerability'. Why are some children not damaged by
deprivation, and can we teach these skills to other children, intervene in other
family environments, to inculcate the same strengths? (Anthony, 1974a,
1974b; Garmezy, 1974, 1980; Garmezy *et al.*, 1979; Pearlin and Schooler,
1978; Pines, 1979).

Stress interactions: 'the straw that broke the camel's back'

A leader in the field, Dr Michael Rutter and his colleagues, conducted an
intensive four-year longitudinal study in London's inner city and on the Isle
of Wight to explore the interactive effects between multiple stresses (Rutter,
1979). They enumerated six family variables which were strongly and
significantly associated with child psychiatric disorder: (1) severe marital
discord; (2) low social status; (3) overcrowding or large family size; (4)
paternal criminality; (5) maternal psychiatric disorder; and (6) admission into
the care of the local authority (Rutter, 1979). Families were separated into
groups with only one risk factor, two factors and so on, and children in each
group then were compared for rates of psychiatric disorder.

Surprisingly, children with just one risk factor were no more likely to have
psychiatric disorder than children with no risk factors at all. If an additional
risk factor was added, however, the risk to the child increased four-fold. Four
stresses produced a ten-fold risk. Each additional stress potentiated the effects
of the others, so that 'the combination of chronic stresses provided very much

more than a summation of the effects of the separate stresses considered singly' (Rutter, 1979). These findings refer equally to chronic and acute stresses.

The analogy to families with genetic disease is obvious. Families with a genetically ill person, or individual at risk, live in a state of varying chronic and acute stresses. If they experience only one stress, no major harm is done. But the nature of these disorders precipitates other stresses. Huntington's disease again provides the paradigm of stress interaction: (1) parent or child progressively handicapped and terminally ill; (2) death of parent, child, or sib; (3) child at high risk with all those attendant strains and choices; (4) grand-children possibly at risk; (5) possible psychiatric illness in the parent, certainly intellectual impairment; (6) possible hospitalization of that affected parent; (7) multiple sibs or other relative also possibly affected; (8) lower socio-economic standing because of the downward mobility of those with the illness; (9) disorderly house because the lack of coordination of the patient may make a mess or the homemaker may be the one ill; (10) severe marital discord; (11) explosive and possibly abusive temper outbursts from the patient; (12) financial strain of one or more family members chronically ill and the necessity for saving for possible future illness, and so on. The point is obvious: the genetic factor serves as a single, isolated chronic stress which is there to potentiate any other stress that comes along.

Rutter found that genetic vulnerability enhanced environmental traumata. 'The presence of a genetic predisposition makes it more important – not less so – to do everything possible to improve environmental circumstances.'

The sex and temperament of the child also seems to have a marked effect in determining how disturbed by deprivation the child will become, perhaps through the mediation of other people's responses. If an intervention can be made with those surrounding and responding to the child, including the school, the situation could possibly improve. Eliminating even one stress from the child's home or school might bring the child back to some manageable baseline before he or she is overwhelmed.

Despite the multiplicity of stresses, Rutter still found that a certain proportion of children flourished in high risk environments. This is not to say that they were unmarked by their surroundings, or even necessarily that they had 'positive mental health'. Rather, these children seemed 'immunized' against the worst traumas, and were resilient, well adapted and thriving.

> . . . and the drifts
> Entomb, at last, the small nest where a skull
> Flimsier than an egg, a drumstick like a straw
> Lie like the crushed works of a watch: your child . . .
>
> *Randall Jarrell: Loss*

Since 1966, E. James Anthony, a psychiatrist at Washington's University Medical School, has been following a group of about 300 children at risk for mental illness. He writes: 'Families can be put at risk by the disasters of disability, disease, death, desertion, and divorce, and these risks are intensified by an economic and social impoverishment of living conditions. They can be rendered vulnerable to these detrimental circumstances by particular types of malfunctioning such as poor communication and emotional contact between the family members, lack of routine and organization, and absence of any plan for the future'. Anthony uses disease ecologist Jacques May's metaphor to depict the relationship between risk and vulnerability. May describes three dolls, one of glass, one plastic, one steel, exposed to an equal blow from a hammer. The glass doll shatters instantly; the plastic is permanently mangled and scarred; while the steel doll may be scuffed up a bit but reverberates from the blow with a fine metallic tone. The aim of risk-vulnerability research is to discover a protective coating for the fragile dolls which might stave off further trauma for some time (Anthony, 1974c).

Like Rutter, Anthony has classified commonly encountered risks and stresses under the headings of genetic, reproductive, 'constitutional', developmental, physical, environmental and traumatic. He and his colleagues then devised a system of interventions with 33 matched pairs of high risk offspring of psychotic parents and children of normal parents. Children of psychotic parents are far more likely than their counterparts from non-psychotic parents to develop often severe psychiatric disturbances during childhood, adolescence, or adulthood.

One early finding of the study was that the greater the degree of involvement of the child with the sick parent, the more vulnerable the child. Another clear result in retesting children after a variety of interventions was that the more time people spent with the child, the more likely were specific susceptibilities to be reduced. Of the various interventions tested, insight therapy stressing therapeutic relationships seemed to be the most effective in reducing vulnerability.

Anthony's study also complements Rutter's finding that 'one of the most striking features of . . . multiproblem families is the chaotic state of their patterns of supervision and discipline. Moreover, poor supervision has been one of the common antecedents of delinquency in most investigations' (Anthony, 1974c). Rutter presents data that good parenting, with strict, consistent supervision (not punitive) which could provide children with structure and control in chaotic, uncertain circumstances was highly beneficial in reducing stress and risk.

Not surprisingly, the nature of the parent-child bond was discovered to be a major determinant in providing children with a haven from stress. A warm, supportive, empathic relationship with even one healthy parent, a relationship characterized by 'high warmth and the absence of severe criticism' reduces conduct disorders in children by 50 per cent in even the most discordant, unhappy families. Parenting does not necessarily need to be provided by the biological parents. A warm, harmonious bond with someone outside the immediate family had a substantial effect in Rutter's study in reducing conduct disorders and other psychological evidence of strain (Rutter, 1979).

> These kids have a tough bite on life
>
> *Norman Garmezy*

Norman Garmezy, a professor of psychology at the University of Minnesota, is a pioneer in the field of 'invulnerability' research. In an exhaustive review of a literature whose paucity attests to scientific disregard rather than lack of subjects, Garmezy and colleagues distilled the most salient features of the achieving disadvantaged child (Garmezy, 1980).

(1) 'Survivor' children impress their teachers and clinicians with their social skills. Peers and friends like these responsive, interpersonally sensitive, cooperative, and emotionally stable children.

(2) These children like themselves as well and have a positive sense of self, with a *'sense of personal power rather than powerlessness'*. (Italics mine).

(3) They feel that they exert control over their environment, not that they are run by it. An internal locus of control.

(4) The dominant cognitive style is one of reflectiveness and impulse control, but they also need intellectual stimulation and challenge at school.

(5) Interestingly, an intact family does not seem to be necessary for 'survival'. How mother copes with a fatherless home does have an impact.

(6) The psychological and physical environment of the home matters. The higher achieving children come from homes that are 'less cluttered, less crowded, neater, cleaner, and marked by the presence of more books'.

(7) Parents define their own role clearly in the family as parental. Role relationships are structured and orderly rather than ambiguously 'pseudo-sib'.

(8) Parents are more concerned with their children's education.

(9) Parents permit their children greater autonomy and self-direction, taking into account their interests and goals.

(10) The children seem to have 'at least one adequate identification figure among the significant adults who touch their lives. In turn, achieving youngsters hold a more positive attitude toward adults and authority in general'.

Garmezy summarizes:

> The intriguing point to be made about the findings of these studies is that
> despite the harshness of life that families encounter, some parents appear to be
> able to foster or enhance in their children the confidence, self-control, determi-
> nation, flexibility, and cognitive and social skills that accompany the develop-
> ment of competence and positive adaptation. These appear to be important
> precursors to the establishment of stress-resistance in children.
>
> (*Garmezy, 1980*)

The relevance of these studies to genetic counseling is clear and encouraging. We have a glimpse from this research of the constituents of stress-resis-
tant behavior and we have some evidence that specific interventions can be
useful to 'inoculate' families, and particularly high risk children, against the
most deleterious effects of stress. Some suggestions emerge for genetic
counselors to pursue.

Strengthen parental bonds

A warm, supportive relationship with the mentally healthy parent seemed to
be the best protection high risk children could have, according to risk research
studies. In families with late onset genetic disorders, the healthy parent may
withdraw from the family because of an inability to cope with the illness of a
spouse, resentment if information about the genetic threat was withheld
previous to marriage, guilt over possible consequences to children, anger
over extra burdens, time demands and financial demands, or any one of a
myriad of motivations. Parents may not even realize that they are withdraw-
ing if they become depressed or guilty. A counselor can provide them with
empirical data to demonstrate to them their potential value in staving off the
worst effects of stress for their children. Healthy parents have a specific role
to master, a 'medicine' to provide their children through their own consistency, reliability, warmth and understanding, organization and coherence as
a person, and optimism.

The ill parent should also be encouraged to take an active role for as long as
possible. Parental instincts can mobilize impressive energies for healthy
action. (Witness a recent incident in which a seventy year old woman
profoundly crippled by arthritis snatched her grandson out of his burning bed
and sprinted him out of the house.) There is often a temptation for the ill
parent to regress to chaotic infantalization which is frightening and destructive both for the individual and the family. Maintaining a sense of mature,
parental involvement, as much as they are able, and teaching ill parents that
they, too, have a role in protecting their children (especially if they may have
also passed on a defective gene) can be very restorative for the entire family.

Shore up compensatory bonds with surrogate figures

In situations of chronic high or low grade stress, it is useful to develop an array of individuals who can provide support. This can ease the burden on the primary caretaker. These surrogate figures may be within the extended family, such as grandparents (who are often tremendously important in helping their own children and their spouses, and their grandchildren, and who may need their own parental role bolstered), aunts and uncles, in-laws, cousins or others. They may be teachers, persons at work, worship, or in the community. A useful exercise for family members is to draw up a 'network map' of important relationships. Often there are interesting differences among family members in the extensiveness of the web they construct; these differences may, in turn, be reflected in the level of coping of individual members. Counselors should consider inviting members of the wider supportive net to sessions.

Teach cognitive skills

In high risk studies a good intellect seems to provide some natural protection, perhaps because bright people find it easier spontaneously to be interested in their environment and to generate alternate means of solving problems. Whatever the native endowment, cognitive skills should be taught which will help a person have some mastery over the environment such as verbal ability, reading, math, memory, and problem solving. Teach how to be receptive to environmental stimuli, to screen what is relevant and to use these factors in problem solving. Help improve judgment.

Assist with developing good impulse control

Feeling overwhelmed by small daily events can compound being overwhelmed by serious life problems. Teach mastery over impulses and feelings as well as the joy of 'letting go', the freedom to express feelings without fear, and the satisfaction of knowing one will not 'blow' and feel regretful afterward. Particularly with a late onset disease, it is helpful to work on a person's time perspective and help them develop a reasonable capacity both to indulge and delay gratification.

'Assertiveness training' or improving self-esteem

Many feel ashamed of their families' or their own genetic 'defects', as they perceive them. Make explicit such self-denigrating images and work with the individual either to recognize their inaccuracy or change the behavior which leads to them. Although people may not say they feel damaged or flawed, their actions may lead others to treat them as if they were. Help provide them with a sense of autonomy and efficacy, of responsibility for their own actions and confidence in their ability to succeed on their own resources.

Ecourage realistic optimism

Above all, support or imbue families with some sense of realistic optimism. They are in charge of their own fate – even if that fate is to cope gracefully with a defective gene. It is up to them how they choose to lead their own lives – not be led by powers they experience as beyond their control. Medical science is achieving dramatic advances. If the future is perceived as smaller domains of manageable time, there is always hope down the way.

> Let no flower of the spring pass by us: let us crown ourselves with rosebuds before they be withered.
>
> *Book of Wisdom*

References

Anthony, E. J. (1974a). Introduction: The Syndrome of the Psychologically Vulnerable Child. *In* 'The Child in his Family' (E. J. Anthony and C. Koupernik, Eds), Yearbook of the International Association for Child Psychiatry and Allied Professions, Vol. 3, pp. 3–10. John Wiley and Sons, New York.

Anthony, E. J. (1974b). A Risk-Vulnerability Intervention Model for Children of Psychotic Parents. *In* 'The Child in his Family' (E. J. Anthony and C. Koupernik, Eds), Yearbook of the International Association for Child Psychiatry and Allied Professions, Vol. 3, pp. 99–121. John Wiley and Sons, New York.

Anthony, E. J. (1974c). The Syndrome of the Psychologically Invulnerable Child. *In* 'The Child in his Family (E. J. Anthony and C. Koupernik, Eds), Yearbook of the International Association for Child Psychiatry and Allied Professions, Vol. 3, pp. 529–544. John Wiley and Sons, New York.

Commission for the Control of Huntington's Disease and Its Consequences: Report (1977). Vol. 1: Overview, US Dept. of Health, Education, and Welfare Publication No. (NIH) 78–1501, p. xviii.

Garmezy, N. (1974). The Study of Competence in Children at Risk for Severe Psychopathology. *In* 'The Child in his Family' (E. J. Anthony and C. Koupernik, Eds), Yearbook of the International Association for Child Psychiatry and Allied Professions, Vol. 3, pp. 77–97. John Wiley and Sons, New York.

Garmezy, N. (1980). Children Under Stress: Perspectives on Antecedents and Correlates of Vulnerability and Resistance to Psychopathology. *In* 'Further Explorations in Personality' (R. A. Zucker and A.I. Rabin, Eds). John Wiley and Sons, New York.

Garmezy, N., Masten, A., Nordstrom, L., Ferrarese, M. (1979). The Nature of Competence in Normal and Deviant Children. *In* 'Primary Prevention of Psychopathology', Vol. III, Part I, Ch. 2, Social Competence in Children (M. Whalen Kent and J. E. Rolf, Eds), pp. 23–43. University Press of New England, New Hampshire.

Harper, P. S., Tyler, A., Walker, D. A., Newcombe, R. G., Davies, K. (1979). Huntington's Chorea: The Basis for Long-Term Prevention. *Lancet ii*, 346–349.

Leonard, C. O., Chase, G. A., Childs, B. (1972). Genetic Counseling: A Consumer's View. *New Engl. J. Med.* **287**, 433–439.

McKusick, V. A. (1976). 'Mendelian Inheritance in Man', 4th Edition, pp. 22, 238–240, 271–273, 434–425. The Johns Hopkins University Press, Baltimore.

Pearlin, L. I., Schooler, C. (1978). The Structure of Coping. *J. Health Soc. Behav.* **1**, 2–21.

Pines, M. (1979). Superkids. *Psychology Today*, pp. 53–63.

Rutter, M. (1974). Epidemiological Strategies and Psychiatric Concepts in Research on the Vulnerable Child. *In* 'The Child in his Family' (E. J. Anthony and C. Koupernik, Eds), Yearbook of the International Association for Child Psychiatry and Allied Professions, Vol. 3, pp. 167–179. John Wiley and Sons, New York.

Rutter, M. (1979). Protective Factors in Children's Responses to Stress and Disadvantage. *In* 'Primary Prevention of Psychopathology' (M. Whalen Kent and J. E. Rolf, Eds), Vol. III, Part II, pp. 49–74. University Press of New England, New Hampshire.

Selye, H. (1982). History and Present Status of the Stress Concept. *In* 'Handbook of stress' (L. Goldberger and S. Breznitz, Eds), p. 7. The Free Press, New York.

Weiss, J. M. (1977). Psychological and Behavioral Influences on Gastrointestinal Lesions in Animal Models. *In* 'Psychopathology: Experimental Models' (J. D. Maser and M. E. P. Seligman, Eds), pp. 232–269. W. H. Freeman and Co., San Francisco.

Weiss, J. M. (1980). Coping Behavior: Explaining Behavioral Depression Following Uncontrollable Stressful Events. *Behav. Res. Therapeut.* **18**, 485–504.

Weiss, J. M. (1982). A Model for Neurochemical Study of Depression, presentation before the American Psychological Association.

Wexler, N. S. (1979). Genetic 'Russian Roulette': The Experience of Being 'At Risk' for Huntington's Disease. *In* 'Genetic Counseling: Psychological Dimensions' (S. Kessler, Ed.), pp. 199–220. Academic Press, London and New York.

Wexler, N. S. (1980). Will the Circle be Unbroken?: Sterilizing the Genetically Impaired. *In* 'Genetics and the Law' (A. Milunsky and G. J. Annas, Eds), pp. 313–331. Plenum Press, New York.

10 Infertility

DAVID L. ROSENFELD

Introduction

Involuntary sterility affects 10 to 15 per cent of all couples attempting to achieve a pregnancy. While 30 per cent of all couples will conceive during the first month that pregnancy is desired and 50 per cent within the first 3–4 months, the cumulative pregnancy rate will reach 85–90 per cent by the end of one year (Tietze, 1960). The remaining 10–15 per cent are by definition infertile. The incidence may be higher, however, in many of the less developed countries where tuberculosis is still prevalent and the rates of venereally transmitted diseases are greater.

There is currently also an increased public awareness of infertility and the medical means to treat this problem. The decreased availability of babies for adoption, secondary to the ready availability of abortion, has reduced the other alternative to childlessness. There is also an improved social climate allowing for the discussion of such matters and the dissemination of medical information. Finally, the later age of childbearing in women who are career-oriented may also contribute to an overall decreased fecundability (Schwartz and Mayaux, 1982).

Causes of infertility

The aetiology of infertility may be equally divided between the male and female partner with at least 10 per cent of all infertile couples contributing jointly. Most causes of infertility are relative rather than absolute, suggesting that fertility is unlikely, not impossible. In addition, because of the inherent limitations in studying the reproductive process, certain assigned causes of infertility may in effect be speculative for that particular couple's problems. This might therefore explain the failure to conceive after successful therapy

Psychological Aspects Genetic Counselling

of that condition. Conversely, couples who do conceive after therapy may have done so despite that condition.

Causes of infertility in the male

Infertility in the male can be ascribed to deficiencies in the semen, immunological factors, or problems with insemination.

Abnormalities of the semen

The normal semen analysis depends on the presence of an adequate volume of ejaculate (greater than 0.5 cc), an adequate density of sperm (greater than 20 million sperm per cc), good motility and forward progression in at least 50 per cent of all sperm, and normal mature morphologic development in at least 50 per cent of all sperm (Macleod and Hotchkiss, 1942). Impairments in both morphology and motility are frequently recognized long before there is a decrease in the actual number of sperm. Because a single specimen may not be a true reflection of sperm quality, at least two, and preferably three ejaculates need be examined. A recent viral illness may impair a semen analysis for at least two months. In addition, excessive fatigue, stress or increased exposure to high temperatures (e.g. saunas, a hot bath) may likewise impair the quality of the specimen.

In most instances, the cause of an abnormal sperm count cannot be defined. This reflects our lack of information about spermatogenesis. While an endocrinological evaluation might uncover some men with diminished gonadotropins, hypo- or hyperthyroidism, hyperprolactinaemia or androgen deficiency, these conditions, while treatable, are unfortunately quite infrequent (Nagler, 1982). Elevated FSH (follicle stimulating hormone) levels often reflect irreversible damage to the Sertoli cells or germinal epithelium.

Approximately 10 per cent of all men and some 40 per cent of men with low sperm counts will have a varicocele or varicosed spermatic veins. This is present in the left hemiscrotum in 95 per cent of such men and bilateral in the other 5 per cent (Dubin and Amelar, 1975). While the exact reason for sperm impairment in this condition has not been defined, evidence suggests that an increase in the scrotal temperature may be responsible. There does not appear to be any endocrinological impairment in such men.

Genital tract infections may impair the sperm quality. Mumps orchitis in the post-pubertal male will result in sterility in 20 per cent of these men. Men with evidence of acute or chronic prostatitis or epididymitis may demonstrate an abnormal semen specimen. T-mycoplasma have been demonstrated experimentally to impair sperm function and may be responsible for infertility and habitual abortion (Caffrey and James, 1973).

Certain drugs and toxins may also affect the sperm count. Alcohol, in excessive amounts, can affect spermatogenesis by both a direct toxic effect on the testicle as well as an indirect effect on the hepatic metabolism of steroid hormones. Daily consumption of marijuana in large amounts may also be directly toxic to sperm. Cigarette smoking may likewise impair sperm morphology. Industrial and agricultural chemicals as well as other environmental toxins may interfere with normal spermatogenesis.

Many more men are surviving after the treatment of certain neoplasias. The use of radiation therapy in such men, even when appropriate gonadal shielding is utilized, may cause permanent damage to the germinal epithelial cells, which are very sensitive to low doses (as little as 600 rads) of radiation. Some of the chemotherapeutic agents, specifically the alkylating agents, are similarly toxic to these cells. The damage is infrequently reversible.

Other medications such as the furadantins, used for the treatment of urinary tract infections, azulfidine, used in patients with inflammatory bowel disease and mono amine oxidase inhibitors may likewise affect sperm function. Men who had been exposed *in utero* to diethylstilbesterol may demonstrate abnormalities of spermatogenesis (Gill *et al.*, 1976).

Anatomical factors may also be responsible for impaired reproductive function in the male. Cryptorchism, even when unilateral and corrected prior to puberty, is associated with reproductive dysfunction in 60 per cent of such men (Lipschultz *et al.*, 1976). Testicular torsion (Nagler and De Vere-White, 1983) likewise may cause permanent damage to the contralateral testicle.

Congenital anomalies such as testicular hypoplasia or aplasia and defects in the development of the vas deferens or seminal vesicles may occasionally be detected. Klinefelter's syndrome (47, XXY) is present in 1/500 males. Many of these men lack the other physical stigmata commonly associated with this genetic disorder and present with a complaint of infertility and laboratory findings of azoospermia.

Immunological factors in male infertility

The spermatogonia occupy an immunologically privileged location within the seminiferous tubules. However, sperm-specific antibodies may develop in the male after testicular trauma, infection or sterilization. In most instances, however, there are no reasons for the development of such antibodies. These antibodies may be of the IgG, IgA or IgM class and may be directed specifically to the sperm head, midsection or tail. While these antibodies may be manifest in instances of sperm agglutination or immobilization, they may also affect the sperm's ability to fertilize an oocyte. There is no evidence at present that such men are prone to other autoimmune conditions (Bronson *et al.*, 1983).

Problems with insemination

Congenital anomalies such as hypo- and epispadias, while not affecting sperm quality, may interfere with the deposition of sperm deep within the vagina. Retrograde ejaculation of sperm into the bladder may occur following surgery of the bladder neck or prostatectomy or in men with diabetic neuropathy. These men may note 'dry sex' or orgasm without ejaculation.

Ejaculatory dysfunction may also be secondary to sympathectomy (either surgical or post-traumatic). In such instances, spermatogenesis is similarly impaired because of abnormalities of testicular thermoregulation. Men who have undergone lymphadenectomy or perineal resections or men who are taking ganglionic-blocking drugs for hypertension may also develop ejaculatory dysfunction.

Sexual dysfunction may also contribute to infertility. While healthy sperm will survive in the normal preovulatory female reproductive tract for 2–3 days, the likelihood of conception is directly related to the frequency of coitus, with weekly rates of 3–4 optimal. Impotence, premature ejaculation and lack of penetration may occasionally be detected in an infertile male. Hyperprolactinaemia, diabetic neuropathy or hypothyroidism may cause impotency, but emotional factors play the largest role in individuals with erectile dysfunction. Pressure to perform is further aggravated by the infertility problem.

Treatment of the infertile male

The treatment of the infertile male is most often unsatisfactory. Success must be measured in terms of pregnancies and not by improvements in semen parameters. Spontaneous pregnancy rates in couples where the husband is oligospermic is approximately 30 per cent. There is no increase in pregnancy wastage or congenital abnormalities in these pregnancies. Claims for therapeutic benefits must be measured against this rate and few modalities for treating the infertile male will exceed this when tested in a scientific, prospective, randomized double-blind fashion. Many claims for successful treatment of male infertility with a variety of hormones, vitamins, dietary supplements or surgical procedures have not been adequately validated.

Improvements in reproductive function will occur in these men with genital tract infections when treated with appropriate antibiotics. Likewise, those few men with proven endocrinological impairments such as Kallman's syndrome (hypogonadotropic hypogonadism with anosmia) or thyroid dysfunction will often benefit from appropriate endocrine therapy. High ligation of the spermatic vein in men with varicoceles appears to improve reproductive function in some men with varicoceles. Men with immunological causes of infertility may demonstrate a spontaneous cure and pregnancies do occasionally occur from such men even without the disappearance of the antibodies. Immunosuppression with synthetic corticosteroids has been suggested, but reports of successful therapy in such men at the present time are anecdotal.

The use of artificial insemination by husband (AIH) is useful in men whose ejaculate is less than 0.5 cc and in men who experience ejaculatory sexual dysfunction, and in men with congenital abnormalities of the penis. Artificial insemination by donor (AID) may be offered to couples when the male partner is azoospermic or otherwise refractory to therapy. An estimated 20 000 pregnancies per year are achieved in the United States by this technique (Beck, 1979).

Both the husband and the wife must agree with and be fully comfortable with the decision to use donor sperm. Anonymity of both the donor and the couple is mandatory. Prospective donors should be screened thoroughly for familial disorders, illness, venereal disease, education and motivation. Semen analysis, blood chemistry, semen culture, immunological studies and karyotypes are performed on all prospective donors. Fresh sperm is preferred to frozen sperm because of the higher pregnancy rates. The donor is selected for the particular couple based on race, physical appearance, and when possible, ethnic and religious background and blood type.

Pregnancy rates approach 80 per cent in such couples, failures being attributed to factors causing female infertility and to a lack of persistence on the part of the patient. While the majority of pregnancies will occur within the first four cycles, occasionally patients will take at least one year to conceive. Success rates are lower in older patients (Schwartz and Mayaux, 1982).

Causes of female infertility

Infertility in the female may be due to disorders of insemination, ovulation or reproductive organs.

Disorders of insemination

Disorders of insemination are best identified with a post coital test. The female partner is examined several hours after intercourse during the immediate preovulatory phase of the menstrual cycle. The cervical mucus is observed for its abundance, clarity, lack of white blood cells and spinnbarkert (stretchability). The number of active, motile sperm are counted. More than 20 active sperm per high powered microscopic field represents an excellent test of insemination, while less than five sperm suggests a problem with insemination. To insure that this test is done at the time of ovulation, when the cervical mucus production, under the influence of high midcycle estrogen levels, is optimal, serial testing may be necessary. The patient is monitored throughout the cycle with a basal body temperature chart to permit retrospective assessment of the time of ovulation.

While sexual dysfunction is an infrequent cause of female infertility, occasionally severe vaginismus may prevent adequate penile penetration. Such patients are invariably unable to undergo an office vaginal examination, a sign that this might be a contributory factor. Developmental anomalies of the vagina are rare and when present are associated with an absence of menses.

Abnormalities of the uterine cervix or cervical mucus may be responsible for 5–10 per cent of female infertility. Congenital absence of the cervix is quite rare and presents with amenorrhoea, cyclic pelvic pain and eventually haematometra. Hysterectomy is most often recommended in these patients. While retrospective studies have failed to demonstrate an association between cone biopsy or cervical cauterization and subsequent sterility, such patients are occasionally seen who have destruction of cervical function, by prior invasive procedures.

Daughters of mothers who took diethylstilboesterol during pregnancy often have abnormalities of the cervix, both histologically and anatomically. Cervical ectropion, the presence of columnar epithelium in the portico vaginalis of the cervix is encountered frequently in diethylstilboesterol-exposed women. Gross structural abnormalities of the cervix include transverse ridges, hoods, protuberances, pseudopolyps, collars and hypoplasia are present in a majority of these women. These changes reflect a failure of the urogenital sinus to develop the fornices and portico vaginalis by the normal local proliferation and central cavitation of the cervical–vaginal junction. These histological and structural abnormalities appear to regress with ageing. Hysterosalpingography has also demonstrated a significantly smaller endometrial cavity area, upper uterine segment and endocervical canal. While the infertility rate does not appear to be higher in this group of women, there does seem to be an increase in ovulatory dysfunction, dysmenorrhoea, ectopic pregnancy, miscarriage, incompetent cervix with second trimester pregnancy loss and premature births in such women (Siegler et al., 1979).

The cardinal rule in managing the diethylstilboesterol-exposed woman is to avoid unnecessary intervention. Locally destructive methods such as cauterization, cryosurgery, conization and excision have resulted in permanent and significant physical damage and sterility. While these abnormalities may occasionally cause impairment of cervical mucus production or anatomical abnormalities preventing normal insemination, most of these women will eventually conceive without treatment (Rosenfeld and Bronson, 1980).

Chronic cervical infections may prevent adequate cervical mucus production and subsequent sperm storage and transport. The endocervical crypts, at midcycle, when healthy, provide a reservoir for sperm storage and release for at least two days following coitus. Infection may impair the physiological production of healthy cervical mucus. In addition, microorganisms may directly affect the sperm. Women with cystic fibrosis will have severe impairment of cervical mucus production.

Sperm antibodies may also be present in the female serum and reproductive tract. These antibodies may be of the IgG, IgM or IgA classes and specifically directed against the sperm head, midpiece or tail. This may interfere not only with sperm transport but also with fertilization itself. There is also recent evidence that women with such allergies, when pregnant, are more prone to miscarriage (Scott, 1982). The incidence of immunological infertility is estimated to be about 5 per cent of all infertile couples and can best be detected through tests which directly identify the presence of antibodies on the sperm (Bronson et al., 1981). The aetiology of such antibodies has not been determined.

Other instances of poor quality cervical mucus can be identified with serial post coital testing and confirmed with mucus penetration testing in the laboratory. Quite frequently, however, no cause of the mucus impairment can be identified.

Treatment of disorders of insemination

In those instances of sexual dysfunction or cervical anatomical variations, AIH can be performed with good results. The use of intrauterine insemination as a means of bypassing a defective cervix has been utilized but with poor results. The importance of the cervical environment for sperm capacitation must be emphasized. Seminal plasma prostaglandins, in addition, cause intense uterospasm and pain.

Treatment of cervical infection with antibiotics should be attempted before potentially destructive cervical cauterization techniques are utilized. The latter on occasion may contribute to irreversible cervical scarring and stenosis. The husband should be simultaneously treated with antibiotics since he most likely harbors the same microorganisms.

The use of low doses of oestrogens given orally prior to ovulation may enhance cervical mucus production and facilitate conception. The overall prognosis, however, for true cervical factor infertility is poor with pregnancy rates in the 20 per cent range (Scott *et al.*, 1976).

Recent evidence has suggested a role for low dose long term corticosteroids for the treatment of immunological infertility. There is no good prospective evidence as yet supporting this contention.

Disorders of ovulation

Disorders of ovulation may occur in approximately 25–40 per cent of cases of female infertility. Ovulation may either be totally absent, irregular, or abnormal. Ovulation is monitored with a daily temperature chart. There is a thermal rise after ovulation due to the hormone progesterone, which is produced by the corpus luteum. Progesterone levels can be measured directly in the blood and levels above 3 ng/ml confirm ovulation. There is disagreement, however, as to the significance of the absolute progesterone level and the normality of ovulation (Rosenfeld *et al.*, 1980).

Under the influence of progesterone, the oestrogen–primed endometrium will undergo specific, daily functional changes in preparation for nourishment and implantation of the fertilized egg. An endometrial biopsy is useful in detecting not only endometrial disease states which could interfere with implantation (i.e. endometritis, endometrial tuberculosis, polyps, hyperplasia, synechiae or myomata) but also assessing the cumulative effect of progesterone and therefore the corpus luteum itself.

An endocrine evaluation should be done prior to consideration of therapy in patients who are demonstrated to have abnormalities of ovulation. While thyroid disease is an infrequent cause of menstrual dysfunction, a serum TSH and T_4 should be performed routinely. Women who have evidence of hypoestrogenism based on vaginal cytology, absent cervical mucus, or failure to menstruate after progestin challenge should have gonadotropins (FSH and LH) evaluated. Elevated values are indicative of ovarian failure, almost invariably irreversible. Ovarian failure may be secondary to chromosomal abnormalities (e.g. gonadal dysgenesis, Turner's syndrome) cancer chemotherapy (alkylating agents or radiotherapy), viral or immunological disorders (Schmidt's syndrome) or idiopathic (premature atresia).

Low gonadotropins in association with a hypoestrogenic state may be associated with hypothalamic dysfunction secondary to weight loss, rigorous exercise, stress or chronic illness. Such conditions often resolve spontaneously (Jewelewicz, 1976). Rarely, pituitary infarction during parturition may result in a hypogonadotropic state (Sheehan's syndrome).

Elevations of prolactin may be noted in approximately 20 per cent of women with ovulatory dysfunction. Forty per cent of these women may have evidence of inappropriate lactation (galactorrhoea). While hyperprolactinaemia may be seconary to elevated TRH levels in hypothyroidism, chest trauma or certain medications (e.g. phenothiazines), most cases are secondary to pituitary disease. Benign prolactin-secreting chromophobe adenomas may be detected within the pituitary gland in nearly 50 per cent of such patients by computerized tomography. There is a correlation between tumour size and prolactin level. Most tumours are less than 10 mm in diameter. The natural history of such tumours is not fully understood as yet, but rapid growth, occasionally with compression of the optic chiasma resulting in temporal hemianopia, is quite infrequent. Occasional spontaneous regression of such tumours has been observed (Kleinberg *et al.*, 1977). While hyperprolactinaemia will interfere directly with follicular maturation, anovulation in such patients is most likely secondary to disturbance of the hypothalamic-pituitary axis.

Menstrual dysfunction may be found in association with certain hyperandrogenic states. Hormonally active ovarian and adrenal tumours, though rare, will interfere with ovulation. Polycystic ovarian disease (Stein-Leventhal syndrome) implies a chronic anovulatory state characterized by menstrual irregularity, obesity, hirsutism, acne and infertility. Oestrogen production is high in such patients and accounts for their propensity towards endometrial hyperplasia and occasionally endometrial carcinoma. The elevated oestrogens are usually oestrone and result from peripheral conversion of both adrenal and ovarian androgens in adipocytes. The oestrogen will have a dichotomous effect on the pituitary gland enhancing LH production and a diminishing FSH production. While the insufficient FSH levels retard adequate follicular growth within the ovary, the high LH levels will enhance ovarian stromal androgen production. Hence, the cycle is perpetuated. In addition, high androgen levels within the ovarian microenvironment will further interfere with normal folliculogenesis (McNatty *et al.*, 1975; Goldzieher, 1975).

In certain patients with infertility or habitual abortion, ovulation occurs regularly but abnormally. This is referred to as luteal phase dysfunction. The luteal phase may be short (less than 10 days) or inadequate, as defined by a normal 14 day duration but with an endometrial biopsy indicating a maturational delay of greater than two days on two consecutive biopsies. Luteal phase dysfunction occurs in approximately 3 per cent of patients with infertility or habitual abortion (Jones, 1976).

While hyperprolactinaemia may occasionally cause luteal phase dysfunction, the aetiology of most instances is poorly understood. The corpus luteum is derived from granulosa cells which are luteinized after ovum release. These granulosa cells, which initially form a single layer about the oocyte, proliferate during the preovulatory phase of the cycle under the influence of oestradiol and FSH. Deficiency in FSH production may lead to a diminished number of granulosa cells with subsequent diminished corpus luteum function. Luteal phase dysfunction may thus be viewed primarily as an abnormality of follicular maturation (Strott *et al.*, 1970). Stress may impair gonadotropin production and result in an abnormal luteal phase. Endometriosis has been associated with luteal phase dysfunction.

Treatment of disorders of ovulation

Patients with elevated gonadotropins are refractory to therapy. Cyclic oestrogen replacement therapy is recommended in such young women to prevent osteoporosis. Cyclic progestins should likewise be administered to protect against endometrial cancer. Infrequently, a spontaneous ovulation and conception will occur in such women as a result of spontaneous maturation of a remaining follicle.

Bromergocryptine, a dopamine agonist, is effective in lowering prolactin and inducing ovulation in hyperprolactinaemic women. The elevated levels return promptly upon discontinuation of the medication. In women who have macroadenomas (tumours larger than 10 mm) noted on CT scan, transphenoidal resection of the tumour or radiotherapy is recommended because of the risk of tumour growth under the influence of the oestrogens of pregnancy. *Bromergocryptine* has been utilized successfully and safely, however, during pregnancy in patients with tumour enlargement (Del Pozo *et al.*, 1974). In hypothyroid women, thyroid replacement will result in a rapid decrease in prolactin levels and prompt return of menses.

The 'fertility pill' commonly used to induce ovulation in anovulatory women is Clomiphene citrate (*Clomid*), a nonsteroidal compound that acts as an antioestrogen, by competing with oestrogens for receptor sites. The pituitary gland, thereby falsely recognizing a hypo-oestrogenic state, will release more FSH and thereby induce folliculogenesis. In women with low or normal gonadotropins and prolactin levels, *Clomid* will successfully induce ovulation in 80 per cent of patients with half of these women conceiving. It is occasionally necessary to sequentially increase the dosage, especially in obese women. *Clomid* is less effective in hypo-oestrogenic women in inducing ovulation. Because of its antioestrogenic properties, *Clomid* may interfere with cervical mucus production and subsequent sperm transport in 10 per cent of patients taking the medication. Treatment with supplemental oestrogens is of questionable benefit. The risk of ovarian hyperstimulation or multiple pregnancy on *Clomid* is quite small (Rust *et al.*, 1974).

In those patients unresponsive to *Clomid*, human menopausal gonadotropins (*Pergonal*) (FSH and LH) may be administered to directly stimulate the ovaries. Follicular maturation is monitored by serum oestrogen values and/or ovarian ultrasonography. When oestradiol values approach 100 pg/ml and/or when the follicle reaches approximately 20 mm, ovulation is induced with human chorionic gonadotropin (HCG), simulating the midcycle LH surge, which is suppressed in these patients by the high oestrogen levels.

Pergonal is quite expensive and potentially hazardous. The ovaries are invariably hyperstimulated to some extent. Severe ovarian hyperstimulation may result in massive ovarian enlargement, pain, ovarian torsion or haemorrhage, ascites, pleural effusion, thromboembolism, renal failure and death. Multiple pregnancies occur in 25 per cent of *Pergonal*-induced conceptions and are unrelated to midcycle oestrogen levels. The pregnancy rates, however, in carefully chosen patients are quite high (60–80%) (Schwartz and Jewelewicz, 1981).

The use of gonadotropin releasing hormone (GnRH or LRH) has recently been utilized to induce ovulation. Pregnancies have resulted from this therapy. The medication may be given in a pulsatile fashion through an infusion pump or by intranasal administration. The treatment is experimental and not as yet commercially available.

Treatment of luteal phase dysfunction remains controversial. While those patients with elevated prolactin levels will respond to *Bromergocryptine*, this is a small group. There are no prospective, controlled studies demonstrating a benefit of any specific therapy of luteal phase dysfunction in the euprolactinaemic female. Induction of ovulation with *Clomid*, *Clomid* plus HCG, and *Pergonal*, as well as progestin support of the luteal phase, have all been utilized with variable results.

Disorders of the female reproductive organs

Disorders of the female reproductive tract may be responsible for 25–40 per cent of female infertility. The patient may present with a history suggestive of such problems. This would include prior gynaecologic surgery, appendicitis, pelvic infection, a septic pregnancy, use of an intrauterine device, and complaints of pelvic pain, dysmenorrhoea or dyspareunia.

Hysterography and endoscopy are the two techniques most utilized for evaluation of the female reproductive tract. The use of the Rubin test (CO_2 insufflation) no longer has a place in modern gynaecology.

Hysterosalpingography can be performed with either an oil-based or water-soluble contrast material injected transcervically under fluoroscopic monitoring. The patient need not be anaesthetized, but infrequently analgesia need be administered. While there is a risk of infection on venous injection of contrast material with embolization of the oil-based medium, these events are quite rare. The major limitations of this procedure relate to its ineffectiveness in defining the status of the ovaries or recognizing pelvic adhesions or endometriosis. The advantages are its ease and safety. There is possibly also a therapeutic advantage in that a 15–20 per cent pregnancy rate has been quoted within six months of the procedure (Siegler, 1967).

Endoscopy includes both laparoscopy and hysteroscopy. The former has replaced culdoscopy for visualization of the female reproductive organs. The latter enables the investigator to view the endometrial cavity, thereby negating the criticism of using laparoscopy alone without prior hysterography.

The procedures are done together, frequently in an ambulatory setting, under general anaesthesia with endotracheal intubation and total muscle relaxation. Tubal perfusion is performed at this time using a dilute saline solution of indigo-carmine or methylene blue dye. While these procedures offer greater risk of complication to the patient, such as perforation of an organ, bleeding, infection or anaesthetic complications, the overall complication rate is low (approximately one per thousand procedures). The procedure offers a much more thorough opportunity to evaluate the female reproductive tract with far fewer false positive and false negative findings than hysterography (Seitz and Rosenfeld, 1974).

Uterine factor

Nearly 50 per cent of all women will develop uterine myomata by the completion of their reproductive life span. In the young woman attempting to conceive, myomata may contribute to infertility or pregnancy wastage. While a submucous location would most likely interfere with proper implantation of the trophoblast, and perhaps sperm transport, intramural and subserous fibroids may likewise disturb normal endometrial development and uterine blood flow.

It is not always easy to determine when fibroids are interfering with the reproductive process. In the absence of other causes of infertility of long standing duration, especially in the older woman, myomata must be considered a factor (Wallach, 1972).

Uterine synechiae or scarring, referred to as Asherman's syndrome, most frequently results from an infection following a pregnancy. A curettage is usually performed at that time. The degree of scarring may vary in severity. Synechiae may cause infertility, habitual abortion, placenta accreta, abnormal fetal presentation, pelvic pain, abnormal uterine bleeding or amenorrhoea (March and Israel, 1976).

Uterine anomalies are present in 0.2 per cent of all women and may contribute to habitual abortion or premature birth. These anomalies are secondary to abnormal Mullerian development with either a failure of fusion or resorption of the embryonic uterine septum. While all uterine anomalies may contribute somewhat to reproductive dysfunction, most are not incompatible with normal reproductive outcomes. Reports of term twin pregnancies in a bicornuate uterus exist in the medical literature. The septate uterus is generally believed to interfere most with the developing embryo, either through limitations of growth or an abnormal vascular supply to the placenta (Jones and Jones, 1953).

Tubal factor

The incidence of pelvic inflammatory disease (PID) has increased dramatically to epidemic proportions with an estimated 500 000 to 1 000 000 cases yearly in the United States. An estimated 15 per cent of all women will be sterilized by a single episode of PID and 30 per cent by a subsequent event. While gonococcus has long been recognized as the leading cause of salpingitis, recent studies in Sweden and the United States have implicated chlamydia as a more important agent. A recent survey of infertility patients with documented chronic salpingitis showed that 75 per cent of these women had no known prior history of acute PID. The ability of chlamydia to cause an occult PID has been recognized. The use of the intrauterine device and a younger age at first coitus have also been demonstrated to increase the risk of subsequent salpingitis (Rosenfeld et al., 1983). In parallel with increased incidence of PID has been an increase in the rate of ectopic pregnancies, secondary to prior tubal damage (Bronson, 1977).

Tuberculous salpingitis as a cause of infertility, while uncommon in developed countries, is a leading cause of sterility amongst women in developing nations. Fifty per cent of these women will have coexistent endometrial tuberculosis. A primary site is infrequently found in these patients. Renal tuberculosis may coexist. An endometrial biopsy in the late secretory phase of the cycle may uncover granulomas in the endometrium. Culture or guinea pig inoculation of menstrual blood may likewise uncover this disease. Hysterography is often useful in suspected tuberculosis salpingitis. The tubes appear rigid with tiny diverticuli and a pipe stem appearance. There is often mid-segmental obstruction (Binor, 1982).

Tubal and ovarian adhesions secondary to prior surgery may interfere with egg capture and subsequent transport in the absence of obstruction (Bronson and Wallach, 1977). Endometriosis may likewise affect the tube.

Many women seek reversal of prior sterilization. In the United States, sterilization is the most commonly utilized contraceptive method amongst married women over the age of 30. With the likelihood for the divorce of a young couple marrying in the 1980s approaching 40 per cent, the physician must be cautious in counselling a young patient about sterilization. Amongst women seeking reversal of sterilization, most of these women were sterilized at a younger age than the median age of female sterilization, 70 per cent were being remarried and 70 per cent of these in turn were marrying men who had no biologic children of their own (Gomel, 1980).

Endometriosis

The presence of ectopic endometrial tissue outside the endometrial cavity is strongly associated with infertility. Endometriosis is seldom seen in fertile women, as judged by the infrequency with which it is noted at the time of elective tubal litigation. Endometriosis most often involves the ovaries or the pelvic floor (uterosacral ligaments, rectovaginal septum, cul de sac) and infrequently involves the fallopian tube.

The manner by which endometriosis interferes with the normal reproductive processes remains elusive. Reports of an increase in peritoneal fluid prostaglandin levels have been contradictory. The presence of mast cells acting as phagocytes has been mentioned as have theories on local immune deficiency. Dysfunction of normal tubal physiology as a primary cause of both the endometriosis as well as the infertility may exist.

Endometriosis is in a sense a social disease, in that it is most likely to be found in more affluent populations. The typical patient is somewhat older, well educated, meticulous about her physical appearance and personal habits, often tense and highly motivated. She often complains of pelvic pain, dysmenorrhoea, or dyspareunia. Surprisingly, the severity of the patient's symptoms do not often correlate with the extent of the disease. Endometriosis can be suggested at the time of pelvic examination by nodularity or thickening of the rectovaginal septum or uterosacral ligaments. Laparoscopy is mandatory, however, to confirm the diagnosis (Kistner, 1975).

Treatment of disorders of the female reproductive organs

The pregnancy rate following myomectomy when done for infertility approaches 50 per cent. At least 10 per cent of the patients will require subsequent uterine surgery unrelated to infertility. When the endometrial cavity is entered at the time of myomectomy, a Caesarian section is recommended should the patient conceive and carry to term. Failure to conceive after myomectomy may be secondary to pelvic adhesions which often develop after this procedure or may suggest that the fibroids alone were not responsible for the problem (Malone and Ingersoll, 1975).

Asherman's syndrome is best treated by lysis of intrauterine adhesions under direct vision through the hysteroscope. Post operative oestrogens are administered in high doses for two months to promote endometrial growth and healing. Prophylactic antibiotics should be utilized. A small balloon or an intrauterine device should be left in place for several weeks after surgery to prevent the uterine walls from readhering. The success rate is inversely related to the severity of the problem. In general, however, the prognosis for these patients is quite good (March et al., 1978).

The mere presence of a uterine anomaly is not an indication for metroplasty (uterine unification). The patient must first have demonstrated repetitive pregnancy wastage before this procedure is to be considered, since there is the potential for loss of the uterus, or secondary sterility due to the operation itself. Eighty per cent of these patients, however, will have a successful pregnancy after a metroplasty. A Caesarian section is mandatory in such instances (Rock and Jones, 1977).

Surgical correction of the fallopian tube previously damaged by infection (tuboplasty) is more likely to fail than to succeed. Even with modern microsurgical techniques, fertility rates (live term births) are only about 25 per cent despite an 80–90 per cent tubal patency rate. These figures reflect the permanent scarring and fibrosis of the tubal mucosa and muscularis, thereby interfering with normal tubal physiology. In those women who do conceive, there is a 10–15 per cent risk of tubal ectopic pregnancy. Pelvic sonography and quantitative HCG titers should be done routinely in these patients at six weeks gestation to insure against tubal rupture and to allow conservative tubal repair (Garcia and Mastroianni, 1980).

The pregnancy rates following microsurgical reanastomosis of the previously ligated fallopian tubes depends on the method of sterilization. Use of the clip or ring or the Pomeroy technique generally destroys very little tube. Patency rates approach 100 per cent and pregnancy rates 60 per cent in such patients. The use of unipolar electrocautery, often done through the laparoscope, often destroys large portions of the fallopian tube, making surgery difficult. At least five centimetres of tube should be present in order to perform a tubal reanastomosis. While bipolar coagulation dissipates less thermal energy, the three burn technique commonly utilized virtually destroys all of the fallopian tube. Pregnancy rates following tubal reanastomosis in patients sterilized through laparoscopic techniques are therefore low. Reversal procedures should not be attempted in women who had fimbriectomies or salpingectomies (Jones and Rock, 1978). Laparoscopy should be done prior to attempted reanastomosis in all patients, in order to insure that adequate tubal segments remain (Rosenfeld and Garcia, 1976).

Women who have adnexal adhesions secondary to prior surgical or gynaecologic procedures have a 50–60 per cent pregnancy rate following adhesolysis. This good result reflects an absence of intrinsic tubal damage (Bronson and Wallach, 1977).

The treatment of endometriosis depends on the extent of the disease. While infertile women with endometriosis may conceive without therapy, most will not. The hormonal treatment of endometriosis is most effective in establishing a pregnancy when there are no ovarian or tubal adhesions or ovarian endometriomas. The creation of a temporary pseudomenopausal state with the weak androgen *Danazol* or synthetic progestins such as *Provera* (medroxyprogesterone) or the pseudopregnancy state with high doses of the combined oral contraceptive pill, will contribute to atrophy of the ectopic endometrium. Pregnancy rates in these patients approach 60–70 per cent. In those patient who fail to conceive, the disease will invariably return.

Extirpation of the endometriosis at the time of laparotomy or destruction with electrocautery or laser energy may offer a better prognosis for fertility, especially in patients with more severe disease. Recent evidence suggests that combining hormonal suppressive therapy using *Danazol* pre- and postoperatively may improve the pregnancy rate with 40–50 per cent of patients with severe endometriosis subsequently conceiving. The disease may recur, however, in nearly 30 per cent of those patients who fail to conceive (Hammond and Haney, 1979).

Future considerations

Through the pioneering work of Drs Steptoe and Edwards, the technique of laparoscopic oocyte retrieval, extracorporeal fertilization, and embryo transfer (*in vitro* fertilization) resulted in the birth of baby Louise Brown in Oldham, England, in 1979. Since that time, physicians in England, Australia and the United States have further developed this technique to a stage where a 20 per cent pregnancy rate may be expected for patients who previously had no opportunity whatsoever for conception. Moreover, there does not appear to be any risk to the offspring of such pregnancies. As more physicians participate in this procedure and personal experience expands, it is hoped that pregnancy rates will improve even more (Trounson and Wood, 1981).

Emotional aspects of infertility

The physician caring for the infertile couple must not only provide them with an accurate and thorough evaluation and appropriate treatment but must also recognize and support the emotional problems of involuntary sterility which result in injury to the self-esteem, self-image and sexuality of the infertile couple.

Feelings of body defectiveness, loss of sexual attractiveness and social unworthiness often accompany this diagnosis. Childlessness deviates from social expectation and as such may have serious consequences for mental health simply because of the pressures of social disapproval. Childlessness may be viewed by society as sexual dysfunction with fertility associated with female genital success and male potency. Society views procreation as an essential part of marriage with childlessness signifying social dysfunction and disorganization. All major religious groups emphasize that procreation is a necessary fulfilment of marriage. This is amplified by the Biblical doctrine which enjoins the couple to be 'fruitful and multiply'.

There is also a commonly held belief in the existence of the reproductive drive or parental instinct which requires fulfilment. A woman who has not experienced motherhood may feel she has failed to develop her feminine role. Likewise in the male, failure to procreate may signify a lack of masculinity. Couples often equate parenthood with maturity, unselfishness and lack of social isolation.

Infertile men and women perceive a locus of control over their lives as being external to themselves. Infertility is associated with much personal stress and sexual dissatisfaction. There is a higher suicide rate among childless couples. Nevertheless, there are no prospective studies which indicate that psychological factors are responsible for, rather than a result of, the sterility.

The physician caring for the infertile couple must be aware of the effect of the infertility on the couple's sexuality. It is important that additional pressures upon the couple be avoided. Many couples who are requested to perform a post coital test have great difficulty. Impotency or ejaculatory failure is not uncommon and creates a tense, embarrassing situation for the couple. The physician should forewarn the couple that this could be a problem and that it is common. This knowledge itself may alleviate much anxiety and perhaps improve patient compliance. Production of a semen specimen by masturbation is likewise often stressful for the individual. This is especially true when the specimen has to be collected in the physician's office. The medical personnel caring for these individuals should therefore be sensitive to the patient's feelings.

Sexual dysfunction in addition may frequently arise when a couple is trying to conceive. The concept of lovemaking has been replaced by one of breeding. The sexual act is no longer a pleasure but a chore. Instructions by the physician to have intercourse every other night on schedule creates a most stressful situation, which often results in coital dysfunction and extreme tension between the husband and the wife. In a similar fashion, recommendations for long periods of continence to increase sperm density may also contribute to sexual dysfunction. Such instruction, moreover, is medically unwise, since sperms do age and thereby exhibit impaired function.

Even when couples are not seeing a physician, there is frequently coital dysfunction at the time of ovulation. The couple will often sense the midovulatory phase of the cycle. Fearing repetitive failure, coitus is occasionally avoided so that the couple may have an excuse (i.e. control) for their expected disappointment. Once again, the pressure of the presumed ovulation frequently creates a performance anxiety on the husband's part, with subsequent impotency or ejaculatory failure.

Women who have had previous voluntary pregnancy terminations present an additional problem. They often feel guilty. There is an additional subconscious assumption that they are being punished. While medically it is quite infrequent that voluntary pregnancy termination contributes to subsequent sterility, the patient may be convinced that there is an association.

The initial response to failure to conceive is one of surprise followed by internalized anger. This is amplified by a tremendous feeling of isolation experienced by the infertile couple. Social contacts are avoided. These patients note a feeling of shame and inadequacy which they do not wish to discuss with others. They develop complicated defense mechanisms to help deal with the inquiries of their friends and family.

These couples also use denial as a coping mechanism. This may be reflected by a lack of cooperation during the infertility evaluation. There is a fear that the physician might discover the aetiology of their problem and that this might place individual guilt or blame or create a feeling of finality. These couples may also experience a period of suffering similar to that seen after the death of a beloved one, in this case one that is potential and anonymous. These couples grieve for something that can never be.

The final stage in this process is one of resolution. This is most frequently done with minimization as the coping style. The couple may minimize their desire for biological children or select a lifestyle which offers an alternative to parenthood.

An additional situation concerns the emotional response of the patient following an ectopic pregnancy. The personal loss suffered as the result of a failed pregnancy is further amplified by the loss of an organ, in this case the Fallopian tube. The female is left not only with a feeling of failure but also of body defectiveness and inadequacy. Her anxiety is further amplified by her fear of sterility, birth of a defective child, or the fear of another tubal pregnancy.

Counselling services, as an integral part of an infertility centre, may help couples rework their concepts of sexuality, self-image, and self-esteem, thereby speeding the process of resolution and acceptance (Rosenfeld and Mitchell, 1979). A trained infertility counsellor should work within the infertility clinic as a source of support for the couple. The counsellor should work closely with the physician to provide such services for those patients who are in need. The physicians should encourage patients who would benefit from such support to participate in the counselling services (Rosenfeld and Mitchell, 1979).

References

Beck, W. W. (1979). A Critical Look at the Legal, Ethical and Technical Aspects of Artificial Insemination. *In* 'Modern Trends in Infertility and Conception Control' (E. E. Wallach and R. D. Kempers, Eds), pp. 259–266. Williams and Wilkins Co., Baltimore.

Binor, Z. (1982). Tuberculous Endometritis, *In* 'Current Therapy of Infertility 1982–1983' (C. R. Garcia, Ed.), pp. 153–156. Mosby Co., St. Louis, Missouri.

Bronson, R. A. (1977). Tubal pregnancy and infertility. *Fertil. Steril.* **28**, 221–228.

Bronson, R. A. and Wallach, E. E. (1977). Lysis of periadnexal adhesions for correction of infertility. *Fertil. Steril.* **28**, 613–619.

Bronson, R. A., Cooper, G. and Rosenfeld, D. L. (1981). Membrane-Bound Sperm-Specific Antibodies: Their Role in Infertility. *In* 'Bioregulators of Reproduction', pp. 521–527. Academic Press, London and New York.

Bronson, R. A., Cooper, G., Rosenfeld, D. L., Scholl, G. S. and Birnbach, S. (1983). Correlation between extent of sperm antibody binding in ejaculate and post coital test results. *Fertil. Steril.* (in press).

Caffrey, M. F. P. and James, D. E. O. (1973). T. mycoplasma as a possible cause for reproductive failure. *Nature* **242**, 120–122.

Del Pozo, E., Varga, L., Wyss, H., Tolis, G. and Friesen, H. (1974). Clinical and hormonal response to Bromergocryptine in the galactorrhea syndrome. *J. Clin. Endocrinol. Metal.* **39**, 18–21.

Dubin, L. and Amelar, R. (1975). Varicocelectomy as therapy in male infertility: a study of 504 cases. *J. Urol,* **113**, 640–641.

Garcia, C. R. and Mastroianni, L. M. (1980). Microsurgery for treatment of adnexal disease. *Fertil. Steril.* **34**, 413–424.

Gill, W. B., Schumacher, G. F. B. and Bibbo, M. (1976). Structural and functional abnormalities in the sex organs of male offspring of mothers treated with DES. *J. Reprod. Med.* **16**, 147–153.

Goldzieher, J. W. (1975). Polycystic Ovarian Disease. *In* 'Progress in Infertility' (S. J. Behrman and R. W. Kistner, Eds), pp. 325–344. Little, Brown and Co., Boston.

Gomel, V. (1980). Microsurgical reversal of female sterilization: a reappraisal. *Fertil. Steril.* **33**, 587–591.

Hammond, C. B., Haney, A. F. (1979). Conservative treatment of endometriosis. *In* 'Modern Trends in Infertility and Conception Control' (E. E. Wallach and R. D. Kempers, Eds), pp. 41–53. Williams and Wilkins Co., Baltimore.

Jewelewicz, R. (1976). The diagnosis and treatment of amenorrhea. *Fertil. Steril.* **27**, 1347–1358.

Jones, G. S. (1976). The luteal phase defect. *Fertil. Steril.* **27**, 351–356.

Jones, H. W. Jr. and Jones, G. E. S. (1953). Double uterus as an etiologic factor of repeated abortion, indication for surgical repair. *Am. J. Obstet. Gynecol.* **65**, 325–339.

Jones, H. W. Jr. and Rock, J. A. (1978). On the reanastomosis of fallopian tubes after surgical sterilization. *Fertil. Steril.* **29**, 702–704.

Kistner, R. W. (1975). Endometriosis and infertility. In 'Progress in Infertility' (R. W. Kistner and S. U. Behrman, Eds), 2nd edition, pp. 345–364. Little, Brown and Co., Boston.

Kleinberg, D. L., Noel, G. L. and Frantz, A. G. (1977). Galactorrhea: a study of 235 cases including 48 with pituitary tumors. N. Engl. J. Med. 296, 589–600.

Lipschultz, L. I., Caminas-Torres, R., and Greenspan, C. S. et al. (1976). Testicular function and orchiopexy for unilateral undescended testis. N. Engl. J. Med. 295, 15–18.

MacLeod, J. and Hotchkiss, R. S. (1942). The distribution of spermatozoa and certain chemical constituents in the human ejaculate. J. Urol. 48, 225–229.

Malone, M. J. and Ingersoll, F. M. (1975). Myomectomy in Infertility. In 'Progress in Infertility' (S. J. Behrman and R. W. Kistner, Eds), 2nd edition, pp. 85–90. Little, Brown and Company, Boston.

March, C. M. and Israel, R. (1976). Intrauterine adhesions secondary to elective abortion: hysteroscopic diagnosis and management. Obstet. Gynecol. 48, 422–424.

March, C. M., Israel, R. and March, A. D. (1978). Hysteroscopic management of intrauterine adhesions. Am. J. Obstet. Gynecol. 130, 653–657.

McNatty, K. P., Hunter, W. M., McNeilly, A. S. and Sawers, R. S. (1975). Changes in the concentration of pituitary and steroid hormones in the follicular fluid of graafian follicles throughout the menstrual cycle. J. Endocrinol. 64, 555–571.

Nagler, H. (1982). Endocrinologic Cause of Male Infertility. In 'Aspects of Male Infertility' (DeVere-White, Ed.), pp. 103–110. Williams and Wilkins Co., Baltimore.

Nagler, H. and DeVere-White, R. (1983). Effect of testicular torsion on the contralateral testis. J. Urol. (in press).

Rock, J. A. and Jones, H. W. Jr. (1977). The clinical management of the double uterus. Fertil. Steril. 28, 798–806.

Rosenfeld, D. L. and Bronson, R. A. (1980). Reproductive problems in the DES-exposed female. Obstet. Gynecol. 55, 453–456.

Rosenfeld, D. L. and Garcia, C. R. (1976). Laparoscopy prior to tubal reanastomosis. J. Reprod. Med. 17, 247–248.

Rosenfeld, D. L. and Mitchell, E. (1979). Treating the emotional aspects of infertility: counseling services in an infertility clinic. Am. J. Obstet. Gynecol. 135, 177–180.

Rosenfeld, D. L., Chudow, S. and Bronson, R. A. (1980). Diagnosis of luteal phase inadequacy. Obstet. Gynecol. 56, 193–196.

Rosenfeld, D. L., Seidman, S., Bronson, R. A. and Scholl, G. (1983). Unsuspected chronic pelvic inflammatory disease in the infertile female. Fertil. Steril. (in press).

Rust, C. A., Israel, R. and Mishell, D. R. (1974). An individualized graduated therapeutic regimen for clomiphene citrate. Am. J. Obstet. Gynecol. 120, 785–790.

Schwartz, M. and Jewelewicz, R. (1981). The use of gonadotropins for induction of ovulation. Fertil. Steril. 35, 3–12.

Schwartz, D. and Mayaux, M. J. (1982). Female fecundity as a function of age. N. Engl. J. Med. 306, 404–406.

Scott, J. R. (1982). Immunologic aspects of recurrent spontaneous abortion. Fertil. Steril. 38, 301–302.

Scott, J. Z., Nakamura, R. M. and March, C. et al. (1976). The cervical factor in infertility: diagnosis and treatment. Fertil. Steril. 28, 1289–1294.

Seitz, H. M. and Rosenfeld, D. L. (1974). Endoscopy in the management of infertility. Clin. Obstet. Gynecol. 17, 86–101.

Siegler, A. M. (1967). 'Hysterosalpingography'. Harper and Row, New York.

Siegler, A. M., Wang, C. F. and Friberg, J. (1979). Fertility of the diethylstilbesterol exposed offspring. *Fertil. Steril.* **31**, 601–607.

Strott, C. A., Cargille, C. M. and Ross, G. T. *et al.* (1970). The short luteal phase. *J. Clin. Endocrinol. Metab.* **30**, 246–251.

Tietze, C. (1960). Probability of pregnancy resulting from a single unprotected coitus. *Fertil. Steril.* **11**, 485–488.

Trounson, A. and Wood, C. (1981). Extracorporeal fertilization and embryo transfer. *Clin. Obstet. Gynecol.* **8**, 681–713.

Wallach, E. E. (1972). The uterine factor in infertility. *Fertil. Steril.* **23**, 138–158.

11 Sterilization

PAULA E. HOLLERBACH
DOROTHY L. NORTMAN

Global view

On a global basis, 100 million couples of reproductive age are estimated to be contraceptively sterilized as of 1980, compared with 20 million in 1970. The 100 million figure is predicated largely on an estimated increase in China from 4 million sterilized couples in 1970 to 40 million in 1980. The remaining 60 million of the 100 million sterilized couples are distributed as follows: India, 24 million; the US, 13 million; Europe, 11 million; Latin America, 4·5 million; and the 7·5 million balance, in other parts of the world (Population Information Program, 1981). Thus three countries – China, India, and the United States – with about 40 per cent of the world's population, account for almost 80 per cent of the world's sterilized couples.

This is indeed a very skewed distribution, but the 100 million estimate of voluntarily sterilized couples leads to two striking conclusions: that sterilization is the most popular contraceptive method, practised by one-third of all couples in the world using any type of contraception, compared with 14 per cent in 1970; and that on a global basis, one-eighth of the couples of reproductive age are contraceptively sterilized (Nortman, 1980b).

While a preponderance of the world's sterilized couples live in China or India, their 20 per cent sterilization prevalence rate among couples of reproductive age is not unique. Other countries with a sterilization prevalence rate of this order of magnitude are Costa Rica, El Salvador, Fiji, Hong Kong, Korea (Republic), Panama, Singapore, Sri Lanka, Taiwan, Thailand, the United Kingdom, and the United States; as well as four states in Brazil – Pernambuco, Piaui, Rio Grande do Norte, and Sao Paulo (Nortman, 1980a, 1982). Many other countries with more modest sterilization levels are exhibiting an unmistakable and impressive upward trend. Examples are Colombia (where the prevalence rate doubled from 4 to 8 per cent in two

Psychological Aspects Genetic Counselling

years, from 1976 to 1978), Malaysia, Mexico, the Philippines, and among developed countries, France, and possibly Belgium and the Netherlands. The World Fertility and Contraceptive Prevalence Surveys, as well as the service statistics compiled by government family planning programs (mostly in developing countries) are the primary sources of data on contraceptive knowledge, attitudes, and use. In the developed countries, contraceptive prevalence rates have been high for decades so that interest focuses chiefly on the changing mix of methods; in the developing countries, method mix is an important consideration within the context of enhancing the level of contraceptive practice.

Legal aspects

In the past decade, laws restricting voluntary sterilization have been repealed, liberalized, or ignored. Countries in which legislation explicitly declares voluntary sterilization to be legal include Japan, Panama, the Scandinavian countries, Singapore, some US states and two republics of Yugoslavia. In China, Korea (Republic) and most countries in which laws are derived from common law (which includes India), voluntary sterilization is legal because no law prohibits it. In countries in which the criminal code was once interpreted as applying to voluntary sterilization on the ground of 'serious corporal injury', prosecution of doctors and subjects is now virtually unknown (Population Information Program, 1981).

Existing laws or rulings that forbid sterilization except for eugenic or health grounds are now rarely enforced and are easily circumvented. To abide by the law, sterilizations are typically authorized as being medically indicated. For the most part, new legislation, court decisions, and administrative regulations now recognize the right of mature individuals to request voluntary contraceptive sterilization and to obtain the procedure upon giving informed consent.

Sterilization has not proved to be the panacea for reducing high rates of population growth that some developing countries once thought it might be. India is the outstanding case in point. Although a high proportion of couples said they wanted no more children, and the government campaigned vigorously in the 1960s and up to 1978 to promote sterilization, in fact, the wives of the men who took advantage of the government's free vasectomy program were past their prime reproductive years (Nortman, 1978). India's experience has documented the need to provide a variety of contraceptives suited to the culture of the society and the particular socioeconomic, demographic, and physiological circumstances of the individual client. In the developed world, the increasing prevalence of sterilization is not likely to have much impact on fertility because couples are effective contraceptors of other modern as well as more traditional methods (Nortman, 1980b).

The growing popularity of contraceptive sterilization in various parts of the world reflects an increasing desire to control fertility, the simplification of techniques, greater availability of trained medical personnel to perform the operations, and acting as both cause and consequence, the method's newly acquired status of acceptability, respectability and legality.

Trends in the United States

The increase in contraceptive sterilization in the United States between the 1970 National Fertility Study and the latest available data from the 1976 National Survey of Family Growth is of striking magnitude. For a detailed comparison, special tabulations were obtained from the US National Center for Health Statistics.[1] Whereas in 1970, 17 per cent of the respondents said they were sterilized, 6·2 per cent for non-contraceptive and 10·6 per cent for contraceptive reasons, the comparable figures (unstandardized) in 1976 were 28 per cent, 9·6 per cent, and 18·6 per cent respectively. Moreover, the 75 per cent gain in the proportion contraceptively sterilized is likely to be an understatement since with no deterioration in health conditions during the interval, the reported 55 per cent increase in the proportion non-contraceptively sterilized probably includes respondents who belong in the contraceptively rather than non-contraceptively sterilized category.

As expected, the higher the parity or age, the greater is the proportion sterilized, for whatever reason. What is striking, however, is the prevalence of sterilization. Even at parity 2, one-fourth in 1976 said the couple was contraceptively sterilized (a three-fold increase over 1970), and another 9 per cent reported a non-contraceptive sterilization. As can be seen in Table 11.1, among parity 3 women, almost half (45 per cent) said the couple had been sterilized, 30·6 per cent for contraceptive reasons; and at parity 4 or more, one-half had had a sterilizing operation, and over a third (36·6 per cent) cited contraception as the reason.

Age and parity being highly correlated, the proportions sterilized with increasing age are equally striking. Thus among women aged 25–29, one out of eight couples was contraceptively sterilized in 1976 (a 76 per cent gain over 1970); among women aged 30–34, over one third of the couples were

[1] The authors gratefully acknowledge the assistance of Gerry E. Hendershot, Statistician for the Division of Vital Statistics, National Center for Health Statistics, who provided tabulations from the 1970 National Fertility Study and the 1976 National Survey of Family Growth.

Table 11.1   Proportions sterilized for all reasons and for contraceptive reasons by race, parity, age group, education, and religion: United States, 1970, 1976. (Selected tabulations from the 1970 National Fertility Study and 1976 National Survey of Family Growth produced by the US National Center for Health Statistics)

Group	1970 Per cent Sterilized		1976 Per cent Sterilized	
	All reasons	Contraception	All reasons	Contraception
Total	16·9	10·6	28·2	18·6
Race				
White	16·9	10·5	29·0	19·3
Black	17·9	11·8	21·6	12·7
Parity				
0–2	9·4	4·2	17·6	11·2
3	23·2	16·1	45·3	30·6
4+	32·1	23·2	54·8	36·6
Age				
<25	1·6	1·4	3·9	3·5
25–29	9·2	7·1	16·6	12·5
30–34	20·8	14·7	36·2	26·4
35–39	29·1	18·0	45·4	28·9
40–44	33·1	16·6	49·0	26·4
Education: years				
<12	24·2	14·4	34·3	21·7
12	14·7	9·2	29·0	19·0
13+	13·8	9·3	22·3	15·4
Religion				
Catholic	10·3	5·8	21·8	13·1
Non-Catholic	19·1	12·2	31·6	21·1

sterilized, and over a quarter for contraceptive purposes; and almost half the women older than age 35 but still in the reproductive years reported the couple had undergone a sterilizing operation.

Age for age, and parity for parity, black couples have considerably lower sterilization prevalence rates than white couples. Indeed, although the prevalence between 1970 and 1976 was increasing among blacks as well as whites, the rate of increase was much higher among the latter than the former. Nevertheless, the proportion of black couples sterilized is also impressive, at a level in 1976 of one out of five for all reasons, and one out of eight for contraceptive purposes. Among black women of parity 3, in 1976 almost one-third reported the couple was sterilized, and at parity 4, the proportion was 40 per cent. (A parity-specific breakdown among blacks by reason for the operation is not warranted because of the small sample size.)

As expected, Catholics are less likely to be sterilized than other religious groups but the differences narrowed between 1970 and 1976. Whereas only 10 per cent of Catholic couples were sterilized in 1970 (for any reason), by 1976 the proportion had more than doubled to 21·8 per cent. Corresponding figures for non-Catholics are 19·1 per cent in 1970 and an impressive 31·6 per cent in 1976 (with 21·1 per cent reporting a contraceptive sterilization). Of interest is the finding that among Catholics of parity 3 or more, one quarter said the couple had undergone a contraceptive sterilization.

Educational differences in sterilization prevalence do not support the hypothesis that the method has greater appeal for the better educated. On the contrary, the evidence seems to be in the opposite direction, 22 per cent of respondents with less than 12 years of schooling (high school graduation) having reported a contraceptive sterilization in 1976 compared with 15 per cent among respondents with 13 or more years of schooling. Among women of parity 2 or less, education makes no difference in the proportion contraceptively sterilized, although the less educated report higher proportions sterilized for non-contraceptive reasons. Only among parity 3 women is the expectation realized that the better educated resort more frequently to sterilization, one-third of those with at least some college education in 1976 reporting the procedure compared with one quarter among those with less than high school education.

A final consideration of these data concerns the gender of the contraceptively sterilized spouse. Here education and race made a decided difference. As can be seen in Table 11.2, among respondents with less than 12 years of schooling, the female is usually the sterilized partner, the female to male ratio being more than 2 to 1. At higher educational levels, the male is more frequently the sterilized partner. Among blacks, the male is rarely the sterilized partner, although the differential narrowed from a female to male ratio of 22·5 : 1 in 1970 to 6·4 : 1 in 1976. Among whites, males and females participate equally in procuring the operative procedure. Use of female sterilization is directly related to parity among blacks, and male sterilization is used primarily by low-parity whites who are highly educated. In 1976, one-half of vasectomized white males had 2 or fewer children in comparison to about a third of the sterilized white females. As for religion, from a 43 per cent female excess among Catholics and 15 per cent among non-Catholics in 1970, the female–male contraceptively sterilized ratio declined to 1·05 in 1976, suggesting first, the elimination of religious differentials, and second, almost equal participation by males and females in voluntary sterilization.

Table 11.2   *Female/male ratio among the contraceptively sterilized by race, parity, age group, education, and religion: United States, 1970, 1976. (Selected tabulations from the 1970 National Fertility Study and the 1976 National Survey of Family Growth produced by the US National Center for Health Statistics)*

Group	1970	1976
Total	1·18	1·06
Race		
White	0·99	0·98
Black	22·50	6·40
Parity		
0–2	0·64	0·76
3	0·88	0·96
4+	0·93	1·75
Age		
<25	0·74	2·40
25–29	1·19	0·94
30–34	1·10	1·39
35–39	1·35	0·98
40–44	1·20	0·77
Education: years		
<12	2·43	2·19
12	0·86	0·87
13+	0·74	0·71
Religion		
Catholic	1·43	1·05
Non–Catholic	1·15	1·05

Factors influencing the adoption of sterilization

A variety of factors account for the increased popularity of sterilization in the United States, some associated with fertility trends and others with the increasing acceptability of the method. Over time, fertility expectations in the United States have converged to a two–child family. Dissatisfaction with the side effects of other contraceptive methods, in particular the pill, increased publicity on all forms of sterilization, and information campaigns designed to reduce misconceptions regarding the effects of sterilization on sexual physiology have also promoted adoption of this method. Finally, removal of age and parity restrictions and the development of simpler surgical techniques reducing the expense, surgical involvement and convalescence previously associated with traditional methods of tubal ligation have also promoted greater availability and reliance on sterilization.

A number of studies have investigated the factors considered in the lengthy decision making process leading to method selection (Mumford, 1983). The primary motivating factor is a desire to terminate childbearing, based on economic or emotional considerations, sometimes accompanied by an unwanted last birth, an unplanned pregnancy, and/or high parity. Fear of an unwanted pregnancy rather than the previous birth of an unwanted child is the more important characteristic. The average age and parity of sterilization users differs by country, associated with legal restrictions on availability, differences in the number of children desired, overall contraceptive prevalence, and the mix of methods available. Research based on the 1965 and 1970 US National Fertility Studies (NFS) based on samples of women under age 45, married with husband present have shown that couples waited an average of four years following the birth of the last wanted child before becoming sterilized, and delay time was longer among low-parity couples and couples selecting vasectomy (Bumpass and Presser, 1972).

Secondary factors in the decision to select sterilization are negative attitudes toward temporary female contraceptive methods, concern regarding the effectiveness or long-term side effects of other methods, and reduction in sexual satisfaction associated with other methods. Reported medical problems and contraindications to use of other methods have also been reported. In contrast, the safety, effectiveness, and convenience of sterilization as well as its noninterference with sexual enjoyment are the attributes of sterilization most frequently mentioned in its favour (Houser and Beckman, 1978).

A third factor implicated in the sterilization decision is consultation with trusted friends who also have elected the procedure and from whom detailed information on the procedure as well as possible physical, psychological, and sexual sequelae can be obtained. This applies particularly to vasectomy decision making, in which friends are often cited as the primary source of information on the procedure. The decision for sterilization is usually made as a couple, although considerable discussion and joint decision making are more typically reported in the selection of vasectomy than in the selection of female sterilization (Alder et al., 1981; Mumford, 1983; Reading et al., 1980).

A fourth factor affecting sterilization decisions is the availability of various procedures, dependent upon the medical and family planning infrastructure in a country, and the cost of the method – both money and time costs (costs of the procedure, travel time, and time lost postoperatively), as well as legal age and parity restrictions on availability.

Perceived advantages and disadvantages of sterilization

The safety, effectiveness, and convenience of sterilization as well as its non-interference with sexual enjoyment are the assets of the method most frequently mentioned. Although greater desire and enjoyment of sexuality and greater frequency of intercourse have been reported in many small-scale surveys, data from the 1970 and 1975 NFS did not show an increase in the reported frequency of intercourse among those couples selecting sterilization during the interim period, although typically coital frequency is positively associated with the effectiveness of contraceptives (Trussell and Westoff, 1980). In contrast, irreversibility and required surgical intervention with attendant fear of pain are mentioned as the method's major disadvantages with cost a secondary consideration. Vasectomy is more often selected for its positive aspects and female sterilization for lack of an alternative method; however, substantial proportions of vasectomized men indicate they would accept hypothetical non-permanent male methods rather than vasectomy (Reading *et al.*, 1980).

Another positive attribute of sterilization is the fact that the method is not associated with hormonal changes. Female sterilization is also the only modern method which usually has no effect on menstrual bleeding patterns. One study, including 1025 cases from five institutions in five countries, compared the effects of the laparoscopic occlusive techniques of unipolar electro-coagulation (504 cases) and the tubal Falope ring (521 cases) on subsequent menstrual patterns. After controlling for prior contraceptive use, the two methods were compared on six menstrual characteristics: the regularity of the cycle, cycle length, flow duration, amount of flow, dysmenorrhea, and inter-menstrual bleeding. The majority of women experienced no menstrual pattern changes following sterilization. Approximately 10–50 per cent of the changes in menstrual pattern within six months following sterilization could be attributed to discontinuation of the pill or intrauterine device at the time of sterilization. However, no statistically significant difference was found between the two techniques in terms of the proportion of women who reported changes in any of the menstrual characteristics (Bhiwandiwala *et al.*, 1982).

Preoperative conditions contraindicating vasectomy and sterilization

Conclusions regarding the psychological sequelae and contraindications to male and female sterilization must be drawn carefully, owing to inadequacies in research design and measurement characteristic of many studies. The most frequent problems encountered include failure to obtain pre-operative measures of psychological status, small sample sizes, failure to examine separately the effects of sterilization sought for medical or genetic reasons versus contraceptive reasons, and inattention to possible respondent bias in follow-up studies, which may select for individuals who have experienced problems. This is especially true in studies using mail questionnaires to assess sequelae. As previously noted, various demographic characteristics are associated with the type of procedure selected, such as age, education, parity and religion. These same variables may be associated with reported sequelae or characteristics of individuals less likely to respond to surveys. Variation in the time elapsed since the operation for the evaluation of sequelae and failure to distinguish short-term versus long-term sequelae represent an additional problem, especially since reports of sequelae may vary, depending on the education and age of the recipient and the time elapsing since the operation.

An even more serious problem relates to the absence of a control group to compare with individuals obtaining sterilization, although the appropriate control group may be difficult to identify. Most previous research has examined the sequelae of one type of procedure as assessed by the user. Ideally, longitudinal studies with properly designed control groups (patients undergoing female sterilization, male sterilization, and those using other effective contraceptive methods) with pre- and post-operative measures of attitudes, adjustments, and health status are needed. Moreover, pre- and post-operative measures of the partner not undergoing sterilization would be useful, in order to assess the impact of sterilization on the couple as a unit. A final problem relates to the actual measurement of sequelae which is typically dependent upon self-reports of regret or dissatisfaction, reduced libido or frequency of intercourse, and menstrual problems which may be psychogenic in origin.

Given these methodological considerations, the psychological effects of tubal ligations (excluding hysterectomies which are often medically-indicated), laparoscopy, and mini-laparotomy are reviewed below. Unfortunately, research is still scarce on the latter two techniques which have recently gained considerable popularity. The sequelae of vasectomy, a more thoroughly investigated procedure, is also examined.

In a recent review of the literature, Wortman (1975) suggests a variety of preconditions contraindicating vasectomy. These include:
(1) Young unmarried men with psychological problems.
(2) Hypochondria in relation to other body functions.
(3) Borderline impotency, homosexuality, doubts regarding masculinity.
(4) Request of sterilization during periods of marital stress, including incompatibility with the wife.

(5) Disagreement or coercion by spouse and passive compliance by the partner.

(6) Belief by either partner that vasectomy is a temporary measure that can easily be reversed.

The suggested contraindications to female sterilization are similar to those of vasectomy (Hollerbach, 1979):

(1) Unsatisfied maternal desire.

(2) Presence or history of previous psychiatric illness or sexual maladjustment prior to sterilization.

(3) Marital instability, doubts about marital permanence, negative spouse attitudes toward the effects of sterilization, or manipulation by the spouse to have the operation.

(4) Misconception regarding reversibility and the after-effects of sterilization.

Sequelae of vasectomy

Despite the lengthy list of contraindications, however, for the vast majority of men and women selecting sterilization, there is reported either no change or an improvement in the quality and enjoyment of sexual intercourse or in marital harmony, and no ill health effects.

One large California study, comparing 4385 vasectomized and 13 155 age- and race-matched, non-vasectomized men, concluded that vasectomy was not associated with any adverse health outcome, including arteriosclerosis (Petitti et al., 1982b). Although some previous research had shown that arteriosclerosis may be exacerbated by vasectomy in some species of monkeys, no evidence gathered in prospective or epidemiological studies, indicates this effect in vasectomized men (Linnet et al., 1982). Moreover, no differences were reported in the incidence of cardiovascular disease and its symptoms. Small but significant increases in back and joint pain, and in kidney and bladder infections were reported by the vasectomized men, although these results could be confounded by other factors, such as prostate surgery at the time of vasectomy (Petitti et al., 1982a).

In another follow-up study, of more than 1000 British males one or more years after vasectomy, only 0·2 per cent indicated that their health had deteriorated and 11·4 per cent reported improvement in general health. Surprisingly, 31 per cent of the wives also reported improved general health (Simon Population Trust, 1969).

Moreover, vasectomy does not seem to affect sexual capabilities. Most of the studies so far conducted in developed countries show that the majority of men and their wives reported either no change or an improvement in the quality and enjoyment of sexual intercourse, or in marital harmony, which they attribute to freedom from fear of pregnancy. Research conducted in Great Britain demonstrates that 73 per cent of the men who had vasectomies reported increased enjoyment of sex; 0·5 per cent reported a decline in sexual pleasure (1·5 per cent of the women); the remainder reported no change. Only 0·5 per cent reported a decrease in marital harmony; 57·3 per cent reported a more harmonious marriage, and 42·2 per cent reported no change (Simon Population Trust, 1969). Other studies on the sequelae of vasectomy based on smaller samples of American or Canadian men, similarly conclude that about three-quarters of the men report greater sexual satisfaction and less than 3 per cent report less satisfaction (Ferber et al., 1967; Grindstaff and Ebanks, 1971; Savage, 1972). The majority of couples who cited problems and requested counseling typically had previous histories of marital, sexual, or psychological instability, in particular, divorce or separation since the operation and the manner in which the decision is made are more likely to be associated with sequelae.

Some authors have hypothesized that a need to reduce cognitive dissonance may result in exaggerated reports of satisfaction with the operation or a reported increase in sexual desire. Thus, to the extent that men are concerned with possible deleterious effects of vasectomy on libido, they may tend to overcompensate in their reports of post-operative sequelae. Such an effect would not be found among the husbands of wives undergoing sterilization (Rodgers and Ziegler, 1973), but should apply to sterilized women as well. On the other hand, other authors have attributed post-operative reports of greater sexual desire to a reduction in the fear of unwanted pregnancy. Similarly, this rationale should accrue to women undergoing sterilization as well as the nonsterilized using effective contraceptive methods. Bean and his colleagues (Bean et al., 1980) suggest a third hypothesis, termed the gender-specific hypothesis, attributing different patterns of sexual effects for men and women. The authors hypothesize that the first-effect, termed a compensatory effect, should hold for males but not for females, since men tend to be more preoccupied with sexual ability than females, and hence sterilization might represent a greater threat to them. The authors also hypothesize that reduction in fear of pregnancy may be less prevalent among sterilized women, especially those undergoing hysterectomy, given the greater trauma of female sterilization than male sterilization, which would suppress sexual desire for some time after the actual operation (Bean et al., 1980).

In an attempt to test what might be termed the compensatory, fear of pregnancy, and gender-specific explanations for reported increases in sexual desire among vasectomized males, Bean and his colleagues (1980) assessed self-reports of sexual desire six months following male and female sterilization, gathered on a subsample of 224 American respondents who completed questionnaires from an original sample of 427 respondents on whom information was gathered at the time of the operation and who agreed to participate in the six-month follow-up. The authors concluded that sterilized females are significantly less likely than non-sterilized females to report an increase in sexual desire both among women receiving hysterectomies as well as women receiving tubal ligations; among males, however, no significant differences existed in reported post-operative increases in sexual desires between sterilized men and the husbands of sterilized women. Although the fear of pregnancy explanation may be operating, resulting in increased reports of sexual desire, the effect is not uniform. Similarly, the compensatory effect is rejected, in that it does not explain results for both males and females. With regard to the gender-specific hypothesis, some support is given to the greater surgical trauma of sterilization for women than for men, having a deleterious effect on sexual desire for women, although the lack of a significant difference in sexual desire among women undergoing tubal ligation versus hysterectomy might argue against this particular explanation. The authors conclude that a more plausible underlying explanation relates to the lower degree of marital communication characteristic of women choosing sterilization, in contrast to men selecting vasectomy. Thus, lesser reported increases in sexual desire by sterilized women may reflect their husbands' lack of involvement in family planning, their relative lack of choice in the selection of the procedure, and the quality of their marital relationships.

Sequelae of female sterilization

Reports on the psychological sequelae of female sterilization pertain primarily to the sequelae associated with tubal ligation, with only a few studies focusing on laparoscopy or mini-laparotomy. Conclusions must be drawn carefully, however, given the methodological problems noted in a variety of studies.

Reports on the psychological sequelae of tubal ligation show an overall positive or at least neutral reaction to the procedure, although levels of dissatisfaction are typically higher than those ascertained in surveys of vasectomized males. In a review of 22 studies conducted between 1949 and 1969 of women who had received tubal ligations for contraceptive *and* medical reasons, Schwyhart and Kutner (1973) conclude that psychological measurements of female reaction to sterilization had been limited primarily to self-reports of regret or dissatisfaction (ranging from 1–18 per cent), reduced libido or sexual adjustment (2–25 per cent), and menstrual problems, which are psychogenic (7–45 per cent).

A variety of more recent Western European studies have also examined the marital, sexual, and psychological sequelae of female sterilization, including a number of hospital studies (Black and Sclare, 1968; Cox and Crozier, 1973; Lang and Richardson, 1968; Neill, 1969; Sim et al., 1973; Thompson and Baird, 1968). One additional study focused on all women sterilized in Aberdeen, Scotland in 1951–1952, 1961–1962, and 1961–1972 (Nottage et al., 1977). The socioeconomic status of the women in these European studies are higher than those sampled in the United States, although average age and mean number of children at the time of sterilization are similar.

On the whole, these studies also confirm the positive sequelae generally reported in American studies of female sterilization. Reported improvements in sexual satisfaction ranged from 27–45 per cent of the women, poorer adjustment ranged from 9–16 per cent in most of the studies. Subsequent improvement in marriage was reported by 45–53 per cent of the sample and deterioration by 6·1–7 per cent. With regard to attitudes following the procedure, satisfaction with sterilization was reported by 76–96 per cent of the women sampled in various studies (Black and Sclare, 1968; Neill, 1969; Sim et al., 1973; Thompson and Baird, 1968). Change in life situation (marital dissatisfaction or dissolution, desire for additional children) or postoperative menstrual problems usually underlie regret, and a high proportion of women requesting reversal demonstrate previous psychiatric disturbance or marital problems (Thomson and Templeton, 1978; Winston, 1977).

Thus, the reported effects of tubal ligation and the degree of satisfaction or regret are comparable in studies conducted in the US as well as Western Europe (McEvoy, 1979). Research conducted in developed nations on the reactions of women having received laparoscopy and mini-laparotomy also show a low incidence of regret or dissatisfaction.

Sterilization techniques have been improved in recent years, stimulated by the needs in developing countries. Since female sterilization involves surgery, it is associated with a substantial risk of injury and a small risk of death, even when the newer procedures are employed. The most serious injuries include injury to other organs and excessive bleeding, technical problems, or major anesthetic complications.

Laparoscopy is performed with general anesthesia, as is minilaparotomy which is becoming more widely used as an outpatient procedure. Multinational randomized studies demonstrate small but clinically manageable differences in complication rates between minilaparotomy and laparoscopy (World Health Organization, 1982). Minilaparotomy is preferred, however, because of its simple training and equipment requirements. Minilaparotomy permits tubal occlusion through a small suprapubic incision through which the fallopian tubes are manipulated for ligation or other occlusion techniques.

Follow-up studies conducted on small samples of American women undergoing laparoscopic tubal ligation indicate that over 90 per cent of the women are satisfied with the procedure. Approximately 95 per cent report either no change or an improvement in their sex life and marital relationship following the operation. Feelings of ambivalence or regret following the operation are not associated with post-operative complications but with the reasons for undergoing sterilization. Sterilizations that are motivated by medical or financial reasons are somewhat more likely to be associated with ambivalence or regret, whereas procedures following attainment of desired family size are the least likely to be regretted (Association for Voluntary Sterilization, 1975; Rubinstein et al., 1979). Based on the success of these preliminary studies, the further development of simple, safe, and inexpensive outpatient sterilization techniques seems to provide a highly acceptable method for women who have completed their desired family size.

Sterilization among the genetic counseling population

Among genetic counselees, sterilization, in particular female sterilization, is more frequently elected by couples whose children's risk for a disorder is high or serious and by those who have achieved desired family size, and by non-Catholics (Blumberg, 1974; Emery et al., 1972; Leonard et al., 1972; McCrae et al., 1973). There is some evidence that the carrier rather than non-carrier spouse is more likely to elect sterilization, however, the procedure is rarely elected following positive fetal diagnosis and selective abortion (Blumberg, 1974). Couples who do elect sterilization at that time usually indicate that the emotional strain they have experienced and their unwillingness to undergo amniocentesis again are the primary factors involved in their decision.

Of course, the attitudes and reactions of individuals undergoing sterilization for contraceptive purposes are not necessarily applicable to individuals seeking genetic counseling. Especially in situations where prenatal diagnosis is not possible, risk factors are unacceptably high, or the family has previously failed to have a normal child after amniocentesis, counselees may elect sterilization to free themselves from fears of future abnormal pregnancies. However, they may still desire additional children, and thus elect sterilization with some ambivalence, and are therefore at higher risk of psychological sequelae.

Counseling recommendations

Guidelines regarding the provision of sterilization, based on age or parity considerations, are poor indicators of psychological or physical sequelae, since the research reviewed demonstrates that most problems which do arise subsequent to sterilization preexisted the procedures.

Guidelines for counseling which which might be suggested apply to the provision of information on any contraceptive method. An explanation of the sterilization procedure to be used, physiological implications of sterilization with reference to reproductive anatomy and possible short-term discomfort during the post-operative period; a consideration of possible life circumstances in which a future pregnancy might be desired; and complete understanding of the permanence, possible complications, failure, and the low probability of reversibility associated with method use. Although reversals are increasingly successful, counselors should present information regarding the nature of the reversible procedure and the statistical probability that an attempted reversal will result in pregnancy. As previously indicated, there is no physiological basis for an adverse psychological or sexual response to sterilization and the discomfort involved at the time of operation or in the immediate post-operative period is comparatively minor. However, these aspects should be discussed with prospective users, since they represent their primary concerns. The research previously reviewed also indicates that individuals with certain preconditions such as marital problems or possible marital dissolution, serious psychological or sexual problems or sterilizations involving coercion, may be more likely to regret the sterilization decision, however, the presence of such problems is not likely to be known to counselors.

The vast majority of individuals selecting sterilization previously have discussed the procedure with other users, and such discussion should be encouraged. Information on the procedure itself, possible complications, psychological and sexual effects, and the effectiveness of the method are the aspects most frequently considered and discussed with other users. Since physicians and counselors often supply only a limited amount of information on sterilization to patients, referral to other sources of information or literature is advisable (Mumford, 1983; for further suggestions see Mumford, 1977).

The genetic counseling population is at special risk of possible psychological sequelae subsequent to sterilization, especially in situations when prenatal diagnosis is impossible, risk factors are unacceptably high, or parents have previously failed to have a normal child through prenatal diagnosis by amniocentesis. In these situations, genetic counselees may elect sterilization to free themselves from fears of future abnormal pregnancies, but still desire children. The few studies which are available on use of sterilization by genetic counselees show that sterilization is more frequently used by non-Catholics and by those who have completed their desired family size. Moreover, genetic carriers, those at high risk, and/or those who risk a serious disorder in progeny seem especially likely to seek sterilization.

Special counseling may be required for counselees whose carrier status is uncertain, those who have not achieved their desired family size, and those who desire sterilization concomitant with selective abortion following prenatal diagnosis of a genetic anomaly. In fact, in the latter case, it would be advisable to discourage the combination of both operations and to allow patients time to separate their feelings of disappointment in achieving a normal pregnancy from the desire to terminate childbearing.

Obviously, however, the safety, convenience, and effectiveness of sterilization are its greatest assets and the overwhelming majority of individuals electing sterilization experience no negative psychological or sexual problems but often report an improvement in functioning. These positive attributes of sterilization should also be presented and the decision to elect sterilization should remain with the patient. Satisfaction with any method of contraception is maximized when users have a full understanding of the relative advantages and disadvantages associated with the method used and are allowed to select methods in a free choice situation.

References

Alder, E., Cook, A., Gray, J., Tyrer, G., Warner, P., Bancroft, J., Loudon, N. B. and Loudon, J. (1981). The effects of sterilization: a comparison of sterilized women with the wives of vasectomized men. *Contraception* **23**, 45–54.

Association for Voluntary Sterilization, Inc. (1975). *AVS News*, December, p. 1.

Bean, F. D., Clark, M. P., South, S., Swicegood, G. and Williams, D. (1980). Changes in sexual desire after voluntary sterilization. *Soc. Biol.* **27**, 186–193.

Bhiwandiwala, P., Mumford, S. and Feldblum, P. (1982). Menstrual pattern changes following laparoscopic sterilization: A comparative study of electrocoagulation and the tubal ring in 1025 cases. *J. Reprod. Med.* **27**, 249–255.

Black, W. P. and Sclare, A. B. (1968). Sterilization by tubal ligation – a follow-up study. *J. Obstet. Gynae. Br. Comm.* **75**, 219–224.

Blumberg, B. D. (1974). 'Psychic Sequelae of Selective Abortion'. Unpublished MD thesis, Yale University, New Haven.

Bumpass, L. L. and Presser, H. B. (1972). Contraceptive sterilization in the US: 1965–1970. *Demography* **9**, 531–548.

Cox, M. L. and Crozier, I. M. (1973). Female sterilization: long-term follow-up with particular reference to regret. *J. Reprod. Fertil.* **35**, 624–626.

Emery, A. E. H., Watt, M. S. and Clack, E. R. (1972). The effects of genetic counselling in Duchenne muscular dystrophy. *Clin. Genet.* **3**, 147–150.

Ferber, A. S., Tietze, C. and Lewit, S. (1967). Men with vasectomies: A study of medical, sexual and psychosocial changes. *Psychosom. Med.* **29**, 354–366.

Grindstaff, C. F. and Ebanks, G. E. (1971). Vasectomy as a birth control method. *In* 'Critical Issues in Canadian Society' (C. L. Boydell, C. F. Grindstaff and P. C. Whitehead, Eds), pp. 25–32. Holt, Rinehart, Winston, Toronto.

Hollerbach, P. E. (1979). Parental choice and family planning: the acceptability, use and sequelae of four methods. *In* 'Counseling in Genetics' (Y. E. Hsia, K. Hirschhorn, R. L. Silverberg and L. Godmilow, Eds), pp. 189–222. Alan R. Liss, Inc., New York.

Houser, B. B. and Beckman, L. J. (1978). Examination of contraceptive perceptions and usage among Los Angeles County women. *Contraception* **18**, 7–18.

Lang, L. P. and Richardson, K. D. (1968). The implications of rising female sterilization rate. *J. Obstet. Gynae. Br. Comm.* **75**, 972–975.

Leonard, C. O., Chase, G. A. and Childs, B. (1972). Genetic Counseling: A consumers' view. *N. Engl. J. Med.* **287**, 433–439.

Linnet, L., Møller, N. P., Bernth-Petersen, P., Ehlers, N., Brandslund, I. and Svehag, S. E. (1982). No increase in arteriosclerotic retinopathy or activity in tests for circulating immune complexes five years after vasectomy. *Fertil. Steril.* **37**, 798–806.

McCrae, W. M., Cull, A. M., Burton, L. and Dodge, J. (1973). Cystic Fibrosis: Parents' response to the genetic basis of the disease. *Lancet* **2**, 141–143.

McEvoy, M. (1979). Women's response to a government program: voluntary sterilization in El Salvador. Dissertation submitted for the degree of Doctor of Public Health, Columbia University.

Mumford, S. (1977). 'Vasectomy: The Decision-Making Process'. San Francisco Press, San Francisco.

Mumford, S. (1983). The vasectomy decision-making process. *Studies Fam. Plan.* **14**, 83–88.

Neill, J. G. (1969). A follow-up study of 100 cases of sterilization by tuballigation. *Ulster Med. J.* **38**, 119–122.

Nortman, D. L. (1978). India's new birth rate target: an analysis. *Pop. Dev. Rev.* **4**, 277–312.

Nortman, D. L. (1980a). 'Population and Family Planning Programs: A Compendium of Data Through 1978', 10th edition. A Population Council Factbook. The Population Council, New York.

Nortman, D. L. (1980b). Sterilization and the birth rate. *Studies Fam. Plan.* **11**, 286–300.

Nortman, D. L. (1982). 'Population and Family Planning Programs: A Compendium of Data Through 1981', 11th edition. A Population Council Factbook. The Population Council, New York.

Nottage, B., Hall, M. and Thompson, B. (1977). Social and medical trends in female sterilization in Aberdeen 1951–1972. *J. Biosoc. Sci.* **9**, 487–500.

Petitti, D., Klein, R., Kipp, H., Kahn, W., Siegelaub, A. B. and Friedman, G. D. (1982a). A survey of personal habits, symptoms of illness, and histories of disease in men with and without vasectomies. *Am. J. Pub. Health* **72**, 476–480.

Petitti, D., Klein, R., Kipp, H., Kahn, W., Siegelaub, A. B. and Friedman, G. D. (1982b). Physiologic measures in men with and without vasectomies. *Fertil. Steril.* **37**, 438–440.

Population Information Program (1981). *Population Reports* Series E, No. 6, Vol. IX, No. 2. Johns Hopkins University, Baltimore, MD.

Reading, A. E., Sledmere, C. M. and Newton, J. R. L. (1980). A survey of attitudes towards permanent contraceptive methods. *J. Biosoc. Sci.* **12**, 383–392.

Rodgers, D. A. and Ziegler, F. J. (1973). Psychological reactions to surgical contraception. *In* 'Psychological Perspectives on Population' (J. T. Fawcett, Ed.), pp. 306–326. Basic Books, New York.

Rubinstein, L. M., Benjamin, L. and Kleinkopf, V. (1979). Menstrual patterns and women's attitudes following sterilization by Falope rings. *Fertil. Steril.* **31**, 641–646.

Savage, P. M. (1972). Vasectomy and psychosexual damage. *Health Serv. Res.* **89**, 803–804.

Schwyhart, W. R. and Kutner, S. J. (1973). A reanalysis of female reactions to contraceptive sterilization. *J. Nerv. Ment. Dis.* **156**, 354–370.

Sim, M., Emens, J. M. and Jordan, J. A. (1973). Psychiatric aspects of female sterilization. *Br. Med. J.* **3**, 220–222.

Simon Population Trust. (1969). 'Vasectomy: Follow-up of a Thousand Cases'. Simon Population Trust, Cambridge, England.

Thompson, B. and Baird, D. (1968). Follow-up of 186 sterilized women. *Lancet* **1**, 1023–1027.

Thomson, P. and Templeton, A. (1978). Characteristics of patients requesting reversal of sterilization. *Br. J. Obstet. Gynae.* **85**, 161–164.

Trussell, J. and Westoff, C. (1980). Contraceptive practice and trends in coital frequency. *Fam. Plan. Persp.* **12**, 246–249.

Winston, R. M. (1977). Why 103 women asked for reversal of sterilization. *Br. Med. J.* **2**, 305–307.

World Health Organization. (1982). Minilaparotomy or laparoscopy for sterilization: A multicenter, multinational randomized study. *Am. J. Obstet. Gynecol.* **143**, 645–652.

Wortman, J. (1975). Vasectomy – what are the problems? *Population Reports* Series D, No. 2. George Washington Univ. Med. School, Baltimore, MD.

12 Psychological Aspects of AID

ELIZABETH ALDER

Introduction

There is increasing awareness and concern for the childless, and as medical advances have made it possible for the majority of couples to control their fertility, the minority who are unwillingly infertile press for medical solutions to their problem. For the couple where the female is potentially fertile but the infertility is due to the male, or where the male carries a genetic defect, Artificial Insemination by Donor (AID) is a possible solution. This procedure involves insemination of the female with sperm from an anonymous donor. If conception occurs then the offspring are genetically unrelated to the husband, although he assumes all social and legal responsibility. Thus AID differs from adoption where there is no genetic relationship at all between parents and offspring, and natural conception where the children are the genetic progeny of both parents. Apart from the differences in genetic relationship there are also the different circumstances under which conception takes place. Insemination is normally treated as a medical procedure and is performed immediately preceding ovulation. Every effort is made by the medical team to dissociate the procedure from any resemblance to sexual intercourse and yet there are likely to be sexual implications of this method of conception.

AID has raised moral and legal issues about both the genetic differences and the artificial nature of the insemination, which continue to be debated. AID has been used to help infertile couples since 1909 when a successful insemination of a Philadelphian business man's wife was reported. The Feversham Committee appointed by the UK Parliament in 1960 to inquire into the practice of AID reported unfavourably, but in 1973 a British Medical Association panel under the chairmanship of Sir John Peel was less critical and today the relatively simple technique of artificial insemination is increasingly accepted and practised.

Male infertility

It has been estimated that about ten per cent of marriages are infertile and in about twenty-two per cent of these the infertility is due to the male (Templeton and Penney, 1982). In these twenty-two per cent the majority show azoospermia or oligospermia on repeated seminal analysis and are therefore unlikely to conceive naturally, and a smaller number have a defect of sperm quality, e.g. motility or sperm morphology. Retrograde ejaculation, which occurs in some young diabetics can also prevent conception. There is an increasing number of men who have had vasectomies in a previous marriage but remarry and wish to have children. In all these cases the man is involuntarily infertile and as he cannot genetically father a child himself he may consider the option of artificial insemination by donor. A second group (some seven per cent of a consecutive series of patients requesting AID reported by Kerr and Templeton, 1976) are men carrying a lethal or deleterious gene and who do not wish to risk the possibility that their children might inherit the defect. Their situation may differ psychologically because they feel they *should not* have children whereas the previous groups find they *cannot*.

Present practice

There are at least 24 centres in Britain that offer AID and numbers are increasing in the USA and Europe (Richardson, 1980). In Britain there are both private and National Health Service centres, some of which charge a fee but the geographical distribution is uneven with a high proportion of centres in London. Fresh and frozen semen is used and donors are recruited from a variety of sources. The Royal College of Obstetricians and Gynaecologists (RCOG) published guidelines (RCOG 1979) for centres planning to set up AID centres but there is considerable variation in methods of selection of donors, and selection and counselling of prospective parents.

Psychological implications

There are both legal and ethical problems of AID in common with other areas of modern reproductive technology. In 1979 a leader in the British Medical Journal, perhaps prematurely, considered that the debate about the ethics of AID seemed to have been resolved although the psychological aspects of AID had not been considered, and again in 1982 the *Lancet* called for more psychosocial research. Such studies that have been done on the psychological sequelae of AID have been severely limited by sample selection. No long-term controlled follow-up studies on the children have been reported and the issue of secrecy makes such research difficult to carry out. The sociological aspects are well described by Snowden and Mitchell (1981) who raise many questions which they believe should be widely debated in society. In 1980 a small retrospective study on patients' attitudes to AID was begun by Dr M. Lees and Dr A. Templeton, Department of Obstetrics and Gynaecology, University of Edinburgh and myself funded by the Nuffield Foundation. I had not been previously connected with the Infertility Clinic and carried out in-depth, semi-structured and confidential interviews with 20 wives and 17 husbands who had been treated at the Infertility Clinic, Royal Infirmary of Edinburgh. Much of the background in this chapter comes from these couples and some results of the study will be presented in the final section.

Diagnosis of male infertility

Men who are unknowingly infertile are likely to be married to fertile partners and in these cases AID may be suggested as a solution. A man may not be aware that he carries a deleterious gene when he first marries or perhaps not until the birth of an affected child. The diagnosis of azoospermia or oligospermia may not be preceded by any ill-health or physical abnormality and so first comes to light during sub-fertility investigations. Most couples use contraception during early married life and either deliberately stop using contraception, such as the Pill, or become less consistent in their use of barrier methods when they feel ready to begin a family. With the emphasis now very much on controlling fertility many couples expect to be able to conceive when they want to and about half will conceive within six months of stopping contraception. Western society generally expects children to be planned and a childless couple may be thought to be so by choice. Individual couples vary in the time they are prepared to wait before seeking advice about infertility and in most cases it is the wife who makes the first approach to the family doctor. The media, and in particular television programmes, have made the public more aware of problems of infertility and heredity.

The diagnosis of male sterility may be given by the general practitioner or the hospital doctor either to the husband alone, or to the couple together. The breaking of the critical news may be traumatic in itself and while the option of AID may be presented among other possibilities, the acceptance of the meaning of the medical diagnosis must be the primary concern at this stage. The reaction of both partners is most likely to be shock, followed by denial, anger, guilt and then grief (Menning, 1980; Berger, 1980). In our study the predominant reaction of the wives was grief and mourning for the children they cannot have. This mourning persisted and even those who later conceived by AID still expressed sadness. In a couple who have already lost a child because of a genetic defect and then learn that other children are likely to be affected there must be additional mourning – for the child that died, and for the children they may never have.

In couples who are considering AID because of genetic risks the husband is not infertile, but learns that any children may die or be handicapped. The couple then have to make a decision whether not to bear further children, or take the risk, or to conceive by AID. If both partners are carriers of a rare autosomal recessive trait then they will be aware that they could have normal children with another partner, but in this case the responsibility is shared. There are further problems if one or both of the parents is already handicapped in which case they may or may not know that the handicap is hereditary. There may have been an infant death already or there may be a surviving handicapped child and the parents not only have to come to terms with his continuing survival, but also the prospect of their future sterility.

AID treatment

Donors

The recruitment of donors may be the limiting factor in setting up an AID service. Increased sophistication in methods of semen preservation has improved success rates with frozen semen and this makes supplies of good quality semen easier to organize. Medical students traditionally have been used as donors but their fertility is usually unproven, although sperm penetration of hamster eggs can now be used to assess fertilizing ability. The RCOG suggests that the following criteria be used for the selection of donors: reasonable intelligence; no personal or family history of an inherited disorder as obtained at interview; no personal history of potentially transmissable infection; an acceptable physical appearance; a responsible attitude and good fertility. Snowden and Mitchell (1981) add another dozen or so desirable traits, some of which would not be likely to be considered as heritable traits (e.g. pleasing personality) by geneticists. A 'responsible attitude' may confer a practical advantage to the clinic service rather than any benefit to the offspring. The aim in the Infertility Clinic at the Royal Infirmary of Edinburgh is to match the husband as far as possible for physical characteristics such as hair, eye colour, complexion and build. Social class and level of education are not specifically matched.

There are scientific reasons for believing that some physical characteristics are inherited but the inheritance of psychological characteristics is disputed. The beliefs of the potential parents may be somewhat different. In the

Edinburgh study most couples believed the donors to be medical students but also expressed a desire that the donor should be as much like their husbands as possible. They thought hair and eye colour were important but would have also liked, in an ideal world, such diverse traits as being a good singer, a keen sportsman and having a good temper. Successful couples would describe how relatives would admire the new baby and point out its 'father's' features. Snowden and Mitchell (1981) describe how many couples who wanted a second child asked for the same donor and they suggest that this indicated a deeper significance and that blood ties were considered to be important in making up a family. It may be important to explore the beliefs that the couple hold about inheritance of characteristics when they are considering the option of AID.

Methods of treatment

Most AID centres use both fresh and frozen semen. Though the pregnancy rates appear to be somewhat higher when fresh semen is used, the advantages of using frozen semen are considerable. Not only can sperm banks be set up which can store a wide variety of donor characteristics but semen can be transferred across geographical regions to reduce the chances of subsequent half sibling mating. In France fourteen such banks were operating in 1979 (Le Lannoa et al., 1980). When frozen, semen can retain its fertility for as long as ten years.

AID is most successful if it coincides with ovulation and in some cases menstrual cycles are regulated with clomiphene. The timing of ovulation may be established by using temperature charts, cervical mucus assessment, urinary hormone measurement or by measurement of the LH surge in plasma. All of these methods impose practical and psychological stress on the woman: 24 hour collections of urine are inconvenient, temperature charts unreliable and many women dislike giving daily blood samples. However, infertile women are noted for their cooperation although one of the psychological implications of any infertility treatment is that women become acutely aware of their menstrual cycles and anxiety can disrupt a normal cycle. The clinic procedure obviously varies with different centres but typically the women are asked to attend on the days around mid cycle.

The insemination can be carried out in an outpatient clinic or consulting room either by a doctor or a nurse. One ml of semen is introduced into the cervical canal with a syringe or straw, and after about 20 minutes rest the patient can go home. The whole procedure may seem detached and clinical to the patient and some clinics make great efforts to make the procedure as relaxed and unstressful as possible. However, there may still be psychological implications and Blizzard (1977) vividly describes the insemination of his wife and his own powerful reaction. There is bound to be stress and apprehension which would be present even at a routine Gynaecology clinic. In the Edinburgh study none of the patients thought of it as an erotic experience in any way. In fact the opposite occurred, and half the couples abstained from sexual intercourse on the days of actual insemination. One wife described how the experience of being inseminated in a totally detached clinical atmosphere influenced her own lovemaking with her husband in the same 'missionary position'. There was no preference for male or female, doctor or nurse to do the insemination but they all felt that personal warmth in the clinic was very important. The procedure was perceived by the women as being akin to injections to induce ovulation and indeed was often presented by the medical profession as such.

Success rates

One of the problems of AID is that the success rate may not be very high and the couples must be prepared for the risk of failure. In our study half of the wives thought their chances were greater than even. Younger women under 30 are more likely to conceive and much depends on the accuracy of relating insemination to ovulation. Many clinics discontinue treatments after six months or so, by which time the chances of success have considerably decreased. Those who are unsuccessful may then have to renew attempts to come to terms with their infertility and may benefit from further counselling. There have been no follow-up reports on unsuccessful couples although clearly they need to be considered when evaluating an AID programme.

Selection and counselling of patients

Poyen *et al*. (1980) ask 'is there a right to AID' . In the centre in Marseilles they rejected 8 out of 450 couples who requested AID, mainly on grounds of psychiatric disturbance in the husband. If the doctor considers AID as a medical act then he can apply criteria for contra-indication just as he would with any other medical problem. However, others would argue that AID is a biological technique and there are only requests for AID, not indications.

Current practice

AID centres can adopt one of three possible policies, and these have some similarities with policies towards requests for termination of pregnancy: (1) To accept any request that is made assuming that the request itself is sufficient justification by itself; or (2) Only suitable parents are selected by the doctor or medical team who may decide to exclude couples with severe psychiatric or physical problems or may attempt to follow the Council of Europe's advice to give AID only when 'appropriate' conditions exist for ensuring the welfare of the future child; (3) A 'middle of the road' approach in which all infertile couples are made aware of the possibility of conception by AID and if they respond positively they are then given full factual details and have careful discussion of all aspects of AID. Whereas for legal adoption, agencies are likely only to consider stable married couples there are no such constraints on AID centres. Cohabitees, single women and lesbian couples may all be accepted by some AID centres. Clearly AID counselling for single women or couples who are not conventionally married is an issue of its own and may demand particular experience in this area.

Another contentious area is the question as to who should be involved in the interview and/or selection. Kerr and Rogers (1975) propose two alternatives: (1) The physician interviews and selects his patients but refers any problems to specialists or (2) All prospective parents are considered by a team which could include a psychiatrist, psychologist, social worker, lawyer or clergyman. The practice varies between centres and the need for secrecy often argues for a one-man approach such as recommended by Klopper (1981). An alternative approach is to obtain a social report from a senior social worker who visits the couple at home (Ledward et al., 1976) and it is arguable whether selection and counselling can be combined in one person or may necessitate a team. At St George's Hospital, London, prospective parents are carefully interviewed by a clinical psychologist or clergyman (M. Humphry, personal communication). The interview includes discussion on motivation for parenting and experience of children, views on adoption, the donor, and secrecy and knowledge of AID procedures. Most importantly, they also explore how the couple would cope with the failure of AID – and AID is often the last chance the couple have to have children. In Lyon psychological assistance from a team of two psychologists and a physician can be requested by couples considering AID or who have already begun a course of treatment (Chevret, 1980). Chevret considered that couples who were seeking AID for genetic reasons were especially in need of help because of the closeness to reality of such fantasies as 'In my dreams, I populate the earth with monsters'. They used psychotherapeutic or relaxation techniques which aim to help the couple adjust to their own lives rather than the birth of a child which was the gynaecologist's aim.

Issues in counselling

In some cases couples who request AID already will have had discussions about the psychological aspects of genetic risks or male infertility. However, such opportunities are not universally offered and it may be that a couple request AID without having first discussed and explored their feelings about the circumstances which led to their request. We have seen above that the diagnosis of infertility itself has psychological implications, and that a couple who already have had a child with a genetic defect or who have learned that they are likely to do so, will have had a psychological shock. Several workers (Berger, 1980; Nijs and Rouffa, 1975; Kerr and Rogers, 1975) have suggested that there should be a delay of several months between the diagnosis or interview and AID treatment. This allows time for reconsideration and opportunity for further discussion. Kerr and Rogers (1975) suggest that in selection and counselling an important task will be to ensure that as far as possible the man has come to terms with his own infertility. The wife should accept her husband's infertility and be able to express and deal with her consequent feelings.

The motivation for parenthood cannot be assumed, for fertile or subfertile couples there is a real choice – they may have to go to considerable effort to have children and therefore make a positive decision. While social pressures to bear children have lessened in recent years there are still expectations from relatives and friends. Self-help groups such as the National Association for the Childless (UK) and Resolve (USA) can help a couple to make their decision. Nijs and Rouffa (1975) describe the desire for a child as involving a crisis of identity and the distress and difficulties of infertile couples have been well described by Menning (1980) and Pfeffer and Woollett (1983).

Secrecy is another important issue that will be raised during counselling. Just as in considering adoption, discussing secrecy may reveal conflicts and assumptions about the husband's infertility, attitudes to genetic inheritance and future relationship with the child. While there are academic arguments for more openness the parents themselves may be anxious to keep the circumstances of the child's conception a secret. Manuel et al. (1980) asked seventy-two couples treated by AID how they felt about secrecy. Thirty-two per cent chose absolute secrecy where they told nobody about AID, male infertility, or even the couple's subfertility problem. The majority (seventy-seven per cent) intended to be absolutely secret about AID. Only sixteen couples (twenty-two per cent) said they would tell the child some day that he had been conceived by AID. However, the couples were interviewed before treatment, and as they knew the chances of success were only fifty per cent many postponed the decision about secrecy until later. This last finding suggests that there is a need for continuation of the offer of counselling and perhaps couples need to be helped again post natally.

Sexual and marital problems may be revealed during discussion of any of the aspects of AID so far considered. One of the benefits of counselling should be increased communication and this can generalize from the subject under discussion to other aspects. The relationship of sexuality to procreation is forced to the attention of all infertile couples as indeed it is to those considering sterilization as a means of contraception (Alder *et al.*, 1980). Sexual counselling may be indicated with couples following the diagnosis of infertility, when considering AID or during AID treatment itself.

While counselling may be considered desirable by physicians and psychologists, the patients themselves may not agree. In our study all twenty wives and all but one of the seventeen husbands said they would not have liked to discuss their decision with a counsellor or similar person. They felt it was their own decision, between husband and wife, and that the discussions with the hospital doctors (who were particularly experienced and sympathetic) were all they wanted. They were also worried that discussion with someone else would increase the risk of losing confidentiality and bring in an element of selection of fitness for parenthood.

Follow up studies

There have been few reports of follow up studies of AID patients. Those that have been reported tend to be anecdotal, and based on small self selected samples, usually from private practice (e.g. Jackson and Richardson, 1977). The results are in general favourable, and most couples want to have a second child by AID. The children are physically and mentally normal or above average. No longitudinal studies where the impact of AID on the development of the child or the couple's long-term relationship have been reported. The main reason for this is probably confidentiality. Couples who have conceived successfully often wish to have no further contact with the clinic. If secrecy is very important to them then a high refusal rate is likely and this will bias the results. These difficulties may be overcome with careful recruitment and more openness about AID in the future. There appear to have been no reports on the outcome for unsuccessful couples which would make up about half the population treated with AID.

In a pilot study of patients' attitudes to AID (Alder *et al.*), I interviewed twenty wives and seventeen husbands using a semi-structured interview schedule. Some of the findings have already been discussed in context. This was a small retrospective study but gave considerable insight into the psychological issues of AID and provided feedback to the clinic staff about patients' attitudes to AID procedures. Before marriage, most of the wives had had no idea that their husbands might have a fertility problem, and it was usually the wife who first approached her GP for help. Most couples had heard about AID first from the hospital doctor but the five most recent patients had all heard about AID from television programmes. Adoption had

Table 12.1   Attitudes of wives to fostering and adoption before deciding to try AID

	n = 20	
	Fostering	Adoption
Unacceptable to both husband and wife	11	4
Unacceptable to either husband or wife	2	6
Preferred AID	6	7
Already fostered	1	0
Refused by agency	0	2
On waiting list	0	1

been considered by all the couples but rejected for a variety of reasons (Table 12.1). The discussions of their views about adoption led to consideration of many attitudes and beliefs about infertility and reproduction. For example, one ex-midwife was concerned about the background of babies that were placed for adoption and her main reason for preferring AID was that the genetic stock would be 'sound'. Thus the consideration of adoption revealed her own beliefs about genetic identity.

Most of the husbands were initially in favour of AID, especially those in social class I or II, but the wives were less keen (Table 12.2). These wives said it was because of the anticipated reaction of their husbands but in fact the husbands were much less concerned about the genetic and moral issues and saw AID as possibly the only way they could have a child. Secrecy was extremely important to nearly all the couples (Table 12.3). Most of the husbands did not discuss their infertility problem with anyone other than the hospital doctor and their wife. There was also secrecy about AID and some wives were even anxious that their family doctor should not know of the AID treatment and that it should not be included in their records in the maternity hospital. Secrecy was obviously very important to these couples and calls for more openness by sociologists may well be met with resistance by the couples themselves.

Table 12.2   Social class and initial reaction to the suggestion of AID (Statistical significance calculated using Fisher's exact test)

	Wives (n = 20)		Husbands (n = 17)	
	In favour	Against	In favour	Against
Social class I and II	11	0	8	1
Social class III and IV	5	4	4	4
Sig. of difference	$p < 0.05$		NS	

Table 12.3   Couples' attitudes to secrecy in AID

	Number who would tell anyone else about the infertility problem		Number who would tell a child that he was conceived by AID	
	Wives n = 20	Husbands n = 17	Wives n = 20	Husbands n = 17
Already have	2	1	0	0
Might one day	6	7	3	1
Unsure	5	6	7	2
Never	7	3	10	14

There was some evidence that both the diagnosis of infertility and the treatment of AID had a short-term adverse effect on marital and sexual relationships. Five wives experienced sexual problems for the first time after diagnosis or during AID treatment, and eight couples avoided sexual inter-course altogether during treatment. The husbands did not report impotence following diagnosis but both partners reported some deterioration in their marriage. This suggests that for many couples there was a need for sexual or marital counselling but it was not clear whether this was related to the initial infertility problems or AID treatment itself.

Conclusions

Couples who learn that there is a high risk that any children fathered by the husband may be born with a genetic defect, have to come to terms with a sense of loss and have to consider the options open to them. Similarly, if azoospermia or oligospermia is diagnosed, the husband experiences shock and the prospect of future childlessness. In both these circumstances AID can provide an acceptable solution to the problem of childlessness. However, the initial problems may remain and the birth of a child may not instantly alleviate feelings of loss or guilt by either partner.

Counselling can help the couple to come to terms with their problem, to understand the procedures and implications of AID and to prepare them for their future role as parents. Those that choose not to proceed with AID treatment or who fail to conceive may need further consultation and counsel-ling and have to readjust to their future without children. Among the couples interviewed the desire for secrecy was very strong and this was linked to a wish to appear exactly like other parents. They had all thought out the implications of AID and although AID treatment was found to be stressful they were in favour of AID in general and the majority of the wives would try again if given the chance.

Now that AID is known to a wider public it is likely to be increasingly requested by couples with infertility or genetic problems. The psychological aspects have now been recognized as being as important as the biological techniques in the successful practice of AID.

Acknowledgements

I would like to thank my colleagues John Bancroft, David Richardson, Allan Templeton and Ronan O'Carroll for their helpful comments on the manuscript, and the Nuffield Foundation for their support of the retrospective study.

References

Alder, E. M., Cook, A., Gray, J., Tyrer, G., Warner, P., and Bancroft, J. (1980). The effects of sterilisation: a comparison of sterilised women with the wives of vasectomised men. *Contraception* **23**, 46–54.

Alder, E. M., Templeton, A. A., and Lees, M. M. (in preparation). Patients' attitudes to artificial insemination by donor.

Berger, D. (1980). Couples' reactions to male infertility and donor insemination. *Am. J. Psychiat.* **137**, 1047–1049.

B.M.J., leader (1979). Artificial insemination for all? *Br. Med. J.* **2**, 458.

Blizzard, J. (1977). 'Blizzard and the Holy Ghost'. Peter Owen, London.

Chevret, M. (1980). Problems related to requests for AID and psychological assistance offered to couples. *In* 'Human artificial insemination and semen preservation' (G. David and W. S. Price, Eds), pp. 399–405. Plenum Press, New York.

Jackson, M. and Richardson, D. (1977). The use of fresh and frozen semen and human A.I. *J. Biosoc. Sci.* **9**, 251–262.

Kerr, M. G. and Rogers, C. (1975). Donor insemination. *J. Med. Ethics* **1**, 30–33.

Kerr, M. G. and Templeton, A. (1976). 'Selection and counselling of recipients'. *In* 'Artificial Insemination' (M. Brudenell, A. McLaren, R. Short, M. Symonds, Eds), pp. 80–96. RCOG, London.

Klopper, A. (1981). AID counselling and recruitment of donors. Paper presented at RCOG workshop on artificial insemination by donor, Birmingham.

Lancet editorial (1982). 'Whither Human Donor Insemination in Britain?' *Lancet* (**i**), 545–546.

Ledward, R. S., Crich, J., Sharp, P., Cotton, R. E. and Symonds, E. M. (1976). The establishment of a programme of artificial insemination by donor semen within the National Health Service. *Br. J. Obst. Gynaec.* **83**, 917–920.

Le Lannoa, D., Lobel, B., Chambon, Y. (1980). Sperm banks and donor recruitment in France. *In* 'Human artificial insemination and semen preservation' (G. David and W. S. Price, Eds), pp. 89–94. Plenum Press, New York.

Manuel, C., Chevret, M., and Czyba, J. C. (1980). 'Handling of secrecy by AID couples'. *In* 'Human artificial insemination and semen preservation' (G. David and W. S. Price, Eds), pp. 419–429. Plenum Press, New York.

Menning, B. E. (1980). The emotional needs of infertile couples. *Fertil. Steril.* **34**, 313–319.

Nijs, P. and Rouffa, L. (1975). AID couples: psychological and psychopathological evaluation. *Andrologia* **7**, 187–194.

Pfeffer, N. and Woollett, A. (1983). 'The Experience of Infertility'. Virago Press, London.

Poyen, B., Penochet, J. C., Mattei, A., Choux, M. (1980). Is there a right to AID? *In* 'Human artificial insemination and semen preservation' (G. David and W. S. Price, Eds), pp. 413–417. Plenum Press, New York.

RCOG (1979). Recommendations for centres planning to set-up an AID service.

Richardson, D. (1980). AID and Sperm Banks in Great Britain. *In* 'Human artificial insemination and semen preservation' (G. David and W. S. Price, Eds), pp. 11–14. Plenum Press, New York.

Snowden, R. and Mitchell, G. D. (1981). The Artificial Family. George Allen and Unwin Ltd., London.

Templeton, A. A. and Penney, G. C. (1982). 'The incidence, characteristics and prognosis of patients whose infertility is unexplained. *Fertil. Steril.* **37**, 175–182.

13 The Emotional Implications of Prenatal Diagnosis

BRUCE BLUMBERG

Introduction

During the past fifteen years, prenatal diagnostic procedures have become firmly rooted as standard components of obstetric care. The tremendous speed with which this technology has emerged has thwarted efforts to fully evaluate the psychosocial sequelae of prenatal diagnosis. While several large collaborative studies have assessed the efficacy and safety of mid–trimester ultrasonography and amniocentesis, relatively few investigators have addressed the emotional issues attendant to these procedures. Although methodologic pitfalls have handicapped scientific attempts to evaluate the psychological effects of prenatal diagnosis, these studies have provided some insight into the impact of this new technology upon its intended beneficiaries.

In the simplest sense, participants in the process of prenatal diagnosis are individuals, and this individuality prevents the description of a 'typical' emotional response to the experience of prenatal diagnostic procedures. The recipients of prenatal diagnosis, despite their diversity of personality attributes, are similar in several important respects. Specifically, the state of pregnancy and the spectre of possible pregnancy loss are shared by all individuals presenting for diagnosis. For this reason, it is imperative that the psychological implications of pregnancy and pregnancy loss, the context of prenatal diagnosis, be explored prior to a consideration of the specific emotional aspects of prenatal genetic diagnosis.

Psychodynamics of pregnancy

Pregnancy, especially first pregnancy, frequently has been viewed as a psychobiologic crisis. Pregnancy compels a woman to reconsider her role

Psychological Aspects Genetic Counselling

and self-image. Akin to puberty and menopause, pregnancy confronts the individual with new emotional and adjustive tasks. Consequent disturbances in the psychic equilibrium of the pregravid state commonly present the appearance of significant decompensation. Not surprisingly, a woman's pre-pregnant personality and neurotic predilections strongly influence her response to the biologic changes and psychological challenges of pregnancy. It must be stressed that, in the majority of instances, emotional disturbance is a normal, rather than a pathological, response to pregnancy. In most cases, pregnant women are able to regain a state of equilibrium either spontaneously or with minimal therapy (Bibring and Valenstein, 1976).

While earliest pregnancy is characterized by a narcissistic concern with prominent physiological and anatomical alterations, later pregnancy additionally involves a growing awareness of the fetus as an independent entity. Although this incipient 'infant'–mother relationship develops gradually, quickening (the first appreciation of fetal movement, ordinarily occurring at 16–20 weeks of pregnancy) must be viewed as a milestone in this process (Bibring et al., 1961). Current techniques, allowing initial auscultation of fetal heart sounds by 11–13 menstrual weeks, present the woman with undeniable evidence of fetal life at an earlier stage. As will be discussed later, the visualization of fetal form and movement by sonography or the identification of fetal sex by sonography or amniocentesis can be expected to accelerate even further the process of fetal personification.

The last weeks of pregnancy witness a reemergence of narcissistic interest. At this time, balanced against a woman's concern for the well being of the child-to-be are fears of self-injury posed by delivery itself. As will be noted, amniocentesis may, at an earlier phase of pregnancy, produce similar concerns for fetal safety and fears of maternal pain or injury.

Regrettably little has been written about the emotional adjustment of fathers during pregnancy. While fatherhood may share many of the social and economic implications of motherhood, biological factors certainly play a less direct role in the required adjustment of the expectant father. However, the occasional occurrence of the couvade syndrome (the psychosomatic experience of physical sensations of pregnancy by the father) suggests that pregnancy may bear paternal emotional consequences similar to those observed in the mother. Pregnancy may accentuate paternal self-doubt regarding the ability to provide for the emotional and financial sustenance of the family unit. If an abnormal child is expected (either realistically or not), this insecurity may be exaggerated.

Just as pregnancy challenges prior emotional stability, the conclusion of pregnancy, regardless of its outcome, requires psychological adjustment. Even following an uneventful term delivery, significant post-partum depression is commonly observed. Such depression may represent incomplete resolution of the maturational demands of pregnancy and an incomplete reorganization of psychic equilibrium (Bibring *et al.*, 1961). Other authors have attributed post-partum depression to hormonal influences, physical discomfort, a loss of the focus of narcissism, or guilt produced by fears of harming the infant. This depressive state is characterized by despondency, feelings of inadequacy, self-reproach, irritability, and anxiety, with frequent psychosomatic manifestations in the form of hypochondriasis, anorexia, or sleep disturbance. Although a relationship between post-partum depression and pregravid personality might be anticipated, studies have been inconsistent in demonstrating this expected correlation. Mild depression has been observed to persist in a small subset of mothers for as long as one year following delivery. More severe affective or psychotic disorders are usually related to pregravid psychiatric instability and are observed to follow 1/500–1/1000 deliveries.

The unsuccessful pregnancy

While normal childbirth may produce disturbing psychic sequelae, pregnancy loss or an unfavorable pregnancy outcome clearly is a more traumatic experience. A substantial percentage of women who abort spontaneously do experience depression following their realization of pregnancy loss. Overt psychiatric symptoms are not infrequently observed in women following spontaneous abortion, and, in some such women, protracted psychopathologic reactions may ensue. The frequent appearance of guilt feelings following miscarriage may reflect prior ambivalence about the pregnancy or a sense of physical inadequacy and responsibility for the loss (Simon *et al.*, 1969). Of course, for planned pregnancies, the decision to reproduce will have been guided by a variety of psychological drives (e.g. demonstration of potency, transition to adulthood and independence, competition with one's own parents, etc.). Therefore, for the individual couple, the specific emotional response to spontaneous abortion will depend upon the nature of the psychological needs that have been frustrated.

With loss in later pregnancy, the parents' greater awareness of an independent fetal identity must be considered. Thus, perinatal loss is appropriately viewed as an experience of bereavement (Morris, 1976). The expected phases of grief can be identified in women who have experienced a perinatal loss, and interviews indicate that such women commonly describe feelings of anxiety, loneliness, and guilt. Furthermore, a mother's failure to mourn effectively for her stillborn may later impair her relationship with subsequent children.

The birth of a defective child also may be viewed as a pregnancy loss, since the parents are deprived of the idealized, healthy child who had been expected. In this situation, mourning for this lost normal child is complicated by the adaptational demands posed by the reality of the defective child. Parents who produce a handicapped child are injured in several respects. Imperfections of the child may be regarded as a failure of the parents' narcissistic attempts to reproduce in a child their own favourable qualities. The defective child may be perceived as reflecting the imperfections of the parents, thereby challenging their feelings of self-worth as parents and as human beings. Subsequent rejection of the defective child often produces guilt feelings that conflict sharply with the 'almost irresistible impulse to deny relation to the child' (Solnit and Stark, 1961).

Pregnancy loss, albeit expected and in most cases desired, is also a feature of elective abortion. The psychiatric consequences of elective pregnancy termination have been discussed and debated vigorously in medical publications. Although fraught with contradictory claims, recent literature supports the conclusion that induced abortion is rarely followed by serious psychiatric sequelae except as the rare manifestation of pregravid psychopathology. Nonetheless, transient and self-limited feelings of guilt, depression, self-reproach, or regret are noted in a substantial number of women in the days, weeks, or early months after elective abortion (Blumberg and Golbus, 1975). These disturbing reactions may be attributable to ambivalence regarding the decision to abort; this uncertainty in turn reflects a conflict between the sociobiological drive to achieve motherhood and the various social or psychiatric forces opposing motherhood in a given instance.

Extending the implications of ambivalence, women who undergo pregnancy termination against their own wills, under coercion from mate, family, friends, or physician (as in the case of maternal illness), are at particular risk for untoward emotional sequelae of abortion. Even prior to the advent of prenatal diagnosis, the rubella epidemic of the mid 1960s afforded an opportunity for investigators to study the maternal psychiatric impact of elective abortion indicated by fetal concerns. When performed for either maternal (medical) or fetal indications, therapeutic abortion generally involves the loss of a desired pregnancy, and it therefore is not surprising to discover that as many as two-thirds of women in this situation transiently experience depression, guilt feelings, and/or regret. While depressive symptomatology appears and may be persistent in women aborted on the grounds of rubella infection, an additional sense of guilt is prominent in women aborted as a result of their own ill health (Simon et al., 1967). This latter observation reflects the woman's self-perception of personal imperfection and inadequacy in the fulfilment of the desired maternal role.

It would not be appropriate to consider the emotional consequences of abortion without directing attention to the social milieu within which abortion is performed. Rapidly evolving concepts of the feminine role and society's fluctuating acceptance of induced abortion must influence the emotional responses of women experiencing elective termination of pregnancy. Although non-parallel methodologies prevent a direct comparison of recent and past studies, the literature supports the notion that the emotional trauma attendant to elective abortion has declined over the past two decades. This observation, in large measure, may reflect the improved level of mental health of *applicants* for abortion which has resulted from the relatively recent abolition of legal requirements of ill health (mental or physical) for the performance of a 'therapeutic abortion'.

The emotional impact of prenatal diagnosis

What, then, is the influence of prenatal diagnosis upon the background emotions of pregnancy and the puerperium? Unfortunately, adequate data do not exist to address this question in its entirety. Most studies of the emotional aspects of prenatal diagnosis are handicapped by their retrospective design. It must be recognized that the psychological effects of prenatal assessment may be felt prior to the performance of diagnostic procedures and even, in some cases, prior to conception. In some families, the advent and availability of fetal diagnostic techniques has influenced reproductive attitudes and practices. For example, before the development of an assay for the prenatal diagnosis of Tay-Sachs disease, the *post*natal diagnosis of an infant with this condition usually discouraged further reproduction. Stated more simply, regardless of the number of previous healthy children in a family, an infant with Tay-Sachs disease tended to be the last child conceived by a family (Myrianthopoulos and Aronson, 1966). In contrast, in recent years, many parents in this situation have resorted to amniocentesis rather than limiting their family size.

Prenatal diagnosis has become increasingly relevant as expanding technology has lengthened the list of conditions that can be recognized in the fetus. Along with these scientific advances has been a growing public awareness of genetic diseases and methods for their prevention. Therefore, it is not surprising that many couples are planning prior to conception (by seeking information) for prenatal diagnosis. One study has indicated that 17 per cent of women receiving amniocentesis (with varying indications for the procedure) 'became pregnant *because* they knew that the test was available' (Finley et al., 1977). In another population of amniocentesis candidates (parents of offspring with spina bifida), 28 per cent claimed that the availability of amniocentesis would influence their further reproductive plans (Hsia et al., 1979). The advent of prenatal diagnosis for neural tube defects has particularly benefited families with a high risk of recurrence and those who have already experienced the full burden of a surviving child with spina bifida (Laurence and Morris, 1981). Unfortunately, prenatal diagnostic techniques are not yet applicable to all genetic diseases, and some families have elected to terminate pregnancy after learning that prenatal diagnosis was unavailable (as in the case of cystic fibrosis) or unsuccessful (as in the case of cell culture failure) (Hook and Wiley, 1979).

Few attempts have been made to describe the emotional state during the first trimester in families planning and preparing for prenatal diagnosis. All pregnancies are characterized by fantasies concerning the fetus, its safety, and its destiny. Periods of exaggerated fear of fetal injury or defect are not uncommon. Since families presenting for prenatal diagnosis usually are at an increased risk for a fetal abnormality, very realistic fears accentuate the normal concern for the fetus. It is predictable that families with the prior experience of a defective child would be especially susceptible to such fears. Thus, expectant families with a previous child with trisomy 21 (with a 1 per cent recurrence risk) have been demonstrated to experience greater anxiety than couples seeking amniocentesis for maternal age only (despite a numerically identical 1 per cent recurrence risk) (Beeson and Golbus, 1979). Further threatening the emotional stability of such previously traumatized couples is the reawakening of guilt feelings that originated with the previous birth of an abnormal child (Fletcher, 1972). For some families, this stress is so severe that the new pregnancy, even prior to prenatal diagnosis, proves to be the terminal event in the parents' relationship (Blumberg, 1974).

The psychological aspects of prenatal diagnosis have been better studied in the second trimester. The anxieties experienced by women immediately prior to amniocentesis have been explored by prospective psychometric studies (Astbury and Walters, 1979; Beeson and Golbus, 1979; Fava et al., 1982) and by retrospectively administed questionnaires (Golbus et al., 1974; Robinson et al., 1975; Chervin et al., 1977; Finley et al., 1977; Dixson et al., 1981) or interviews (Silvestre and Fresco, 1980; Dixson et al., 1981). Few women completely deny all concerns prior to amniocentesis. Most women express fears relating to the unknown aspect of the test, the anticipation of pain, the risk of fetal injury or demise, and possible injury to themselves. Of course, most women will admit concern relating to the amniocentesis result and to the difficult decision that might be necessitated by the discovery of a fetal defect. The depression and somatic symptoms that are sometimes exhibited prior to amniocentesis may fade immediately after the successful completion of the procedure or may persist until normal results are made available. Fears of pain, injury, or the unknown may be projected transiently as hostility toward the medical personnel (Fava et al., 1982). It would be anticipated that more invasive diagnostic procedures (e.g. fetoscopy) would generate even higher levels of anxiety, but there are no data to substantiate this speculation.

Not surprisingly, the three to four week period between the performance of amniocentesis and the communication of its result is fraught with anticipatory anxiety for many couples. Marital conflicts frequently are noted at this time. Couples at high risk for (or with the previous experience of) an abnormality are particularly burdened during this phase of prenatal diagnosis (Blumberg et al., 1975; Beeson and Golbus, 1979). When asked to suggest improvements in the amniocentesis procedure, women most frequently recommend shortening of this waiting period. Fears during this stage initially may be focused upon possible fetal injury or miscarriage, but such concerns generally subside within several days after the procedure. In contrast, anxieties relating to the anticipation of test results are magnified as the period of waiting proceeds, and it is not unusual for the counsellor to receive telephone calls from the worried parents at this time.

The psychic stresses of this period are exacerbated by the simultaneous occurrence of quickening in most women. Whereas this physiological event ordinarily ushers in a new developmental phase of pregnancy with cathexis of the fetus as an independent entity (Bibring et al., 1961), this process is often arrested in the woman who has undergone amniocentesis. Recognition of the fetus as a potential child may, to whatever extent possible, be held in abeyance until a test result reveals whether the fetus is indeed a potential child or instead a potential abortus. This suspension of investment in the pregnancy may lead the mother to postpone pregnancy-related behaviour (wearing maternity clothes or taking prenatal vitamins, for example) until a normal diagnostic result assures the continuation of the pregnancy (Beeson and Golbus, 1979). Occasionally, a woman in this situation may go to great lengths in order to deny the reality of fetal existence. Such is the case with a multiparous woman who steadfastly interpreted intra-abdominal sensations as 'gas pains' until two days after the communication of normal amniocentesis results, at which time she was able to admit to herself that she had indeed experienced quickening several weeks earlier.

It is quite common during the diagnostic process for a woman to conceal a pregnancy from her friends, acquaintances, and even family members in order to avoid the potential necessity of explaining an abnormal result or an ensuing selective abortion. In contrast, some women freely discuss their pregnancies and plans for amniocentesis with those around them (Verjaal et al., 1982). This openness may serve the function of recruiting a support system that may be relied upon in the event of an abnormal result (Ashery, 1981).

As previously noted, quickening has long been recognized as a catalyst to the perception of the fetus as an independent entity. Recent technological advances, however, have created a situation in which many pregnant women are presented with tangible and indisputable evidence of fetal existence long before the conscious recognition of fetal activity. With the advent of amplified

'Doppler' auscultation of fetal heart sounds, many women are provided with the opportunity to hear 'baby's heartbeat' as early as 11–13 menstrual weeks.

In a similar fashion, ultrasonography facilitates personification of the fetus. The visual images of fetal anatomy and movement serve to enrich the mother's pre-existing mental imagery of the fetus (Milne and Rich, 1981). It is not uncommon for a sonogram copy to be preserved and cherished as 'baby's first picture'. When performed as an adjunct to amniocentesis, sonography, by promoting an intimate awareness of and attachment to the fetus, may counter parental attempts to maintain emotional distance from the fetus while awaiting amniocentesis results.

Fortunately, in the majority of cases, prenatal studies reveal no abnormalities. For most women, the normal results of diagnostic tests immediately alleviate previous anxieties. However, a smaller number of women continue to experience concerns based upon their uncertainty of the test's accuracy and their persistent fears of delayed miscarriage or fetal injury secondary to amniocentesis (Golbus et al., 1974). In fact, some women continue to harbour fears of occult amniocentesis-induced trauma even after the subsequent delivery of a healthy child. For this reason, some women may adopt a more 'cautious and protective' attitude toward their children as a result of the concerns engendered by prenatal diagnosis (Robinson et al., 1975).

As has been noted, normal results of prenatal studies do not always provide enough reassurance to allay parental concerns. In this context, it is appropriate to consider the unique circumstances of maternal serum alpha-fetoprotein (AFP) screening as a technique of prenatal diagnosis. Maternal serum screening differs from other prenatal diagnostic modalities in several important respects. In contrast to amniocentesis, AFP screening is most often offered to women who are at a low a priori risk for an abnormal result. Furthermore, initial serum screening is a relatively non-invasive procedure with no risk to the fetus. Therefore, the decision to accept serum screening is unlikely to provoke the anxieties that are commonly associated with amniocentesis. However, in approximately 5 per cent of women receiving AFP tests, an elevated level will suddenly and unexpectedly confront the couple with the possibility of a fetal anomaly. Although subsequent diagnostic studies usually indicate that fetal defects were not the cause of the initial elevations, residual parental anxiety may be observed (Fearn et al., 1982). If a persistently elevated AFP level remains unexplained, amniocentesis is offered as a more definitive test. In the small group of women who have declined amniocentesis after reaching this phase of the screening protocol, extreme anxiety has persisted throughout pregnancy and even after the birth of an ostensibly normal child; such women have waited for and dreaded the appearance of some abnormality to explain their aberrant test results (Burton et al., 1982). The stigma of an abnormal initial screening result may be difficult to erase completely.

The abnormal fetus

Although the fear of an abnormal result almost always colours the emotional response to prenatal diagnosis, few families are subjected to the acute trauma imparted by the actual discovery of a fetal defect. The recognition of an unfavourable result triggers an immediate grief response that may be characterized by shock, disbelief, and anger, even in cases in which the *a priori* risk of an adverse outcome had been substantial (for example, the 25 per cent risk of an affected fetus in the case of an autosomal recessive disease) (Fletcher, 1972; Blumberg, 1974; Blumberg *et al.*, 1975; Donnai *et al.*, 1981; Adler and Kushnick, 1982). Previous hopes and expectations are crushed by the sudden revelation of a fetal defect. The medicolegal necessity of a swift decision to continue or terminate the pregnancy further burdens the already traumatized family. Prior abstract abortion attitudes provide little guidance for couples so suddenly entrapped in this moral quandary. Ultimately, the parents' understanding of the specific detected fetal defect is a significant determinant of their course of decision and action.

It is the responsibility of the counsellor to provide the family with a balanced and comprehensive picture of the anticipated clinical abnormality. Couples who have had a prior direct encounter with the discovered disorder, as in the case of a previously affected child, will be influenced strongly by the quality of this earlier experience. When only one member of the couple has faced the disorder previously, as in the case of an affected parental sibling, the intensity of emotion evoked by the fetal anomaly may be dissimilar in the two parents. In this instance, the counsellor must promote empathic dialogue between the two partners in order to close this gap and foster a sense of shared experience.

While the detection of a definite fetal abnormality clearly creates a crisis in the pregnancy, the discovery of an ambiguous or uncertain fetal defect stresses the parents' decision-making abilities to an even greater extent. In some instances, it is impossible to predict the clinical significance of an abnormal test result (e.g. 46,XX/45,XO mosaicism, a *de novo* rearrangement, or an unidentified sonographic detail). In such cases, it is incumbent upon the counsellor to define the entire spectrum of possible clinical outcomes. In view of the ambiguity inherent to this circumstance, the parents are extremely dependent upon the counsellor's objective and subjective interpretation of the available data.

Diagnostic imprecision is an even greater problem for disorders that are only suggested rather than directly detected prenatally. For example, the identification of a male fetus in the pregnancy of a Duchenne muscular dystrophy carrier merely predicts the 50 per cent risk that the fetus will be affected. To a lesser extent, such uncertainty is intrinsic to all procedures relying upon linkage relationships to make a diagnosis. In these situations, however, it is not the counsellor's interpretation of the result but rather the parents' assessment of the pertinent risk and associated burden that will determine the course of decision.

Couples faced with such diagnostic uncertainty will be ambivalent regardless of the course of action taken. Those electing to continue pregnancy must anxiously await the outcome; if an abnormal child is born, the parents may experience guilt for what they regard as a preventable tragedy. If, on the other hand, the parents opt for pregnancy termination, they may be plagued by the lingering suspicion that a normal fetus was aborted. Such couples commonly employ the defensive strategy of convincing themselves that the fetus was indeed abnormal, when, in fact, there is no factual basis for their certainty. If a fetal defect is documented after the abortion, the parents will feel relieved and vindicated in their decision. If an apparently normal fetus is encountered after termination, this reality must be couched in such a way as to avoid an undercutting of parental coping mechanisms.

Relatively few couples have continued pregnancies following the discovery of definite fetal defect; thus, little is known of their emotional state during late pregnancy. Some families who have elected to continue pregnancies after learning of a fetal defect have described the benefits afforded by this opportunity to prepare for the birth of an abnormal child (Golbus *et al.*, 1974), but this assertion may represent cognitive dissonance or a retrospective attempt to justify, in their own minds, the decision to proceed with the pregnancy.

A couple may elect to continue a pregnancy under these circumstances for a variety of reasons. The predicted abnormality may not be severe enough, in the parents' opinion, to warrant abortion (e.g. sex chromosome aneuploidy). Occasionally, pregnancy may be continued despite the recognition of a severe fetal anomaly. This course may be followed by families with deep-rooted anti-abortion attitudes or by women who find themselves emotionally unable to terminate a pregnancy at such a late stage. Insufficient information is available to describe the psychological state of these families during the remainder of pregnancy. It might be expected that the emotions ordinarily associated with the birth of an abnormal child would materialize soon after the decision to proceed with pregnancy. Presumably, by the time of delivery, these parents would have had some opportunity to come to grips with their feelings and to prepare for the many practical demands presented by an abnormal neonate.

Somewhat more is known of the emotional responses of families selecting abortion after a prenatal diagnosis. Post-abortion depression is frequent and often is severe when a fetal abnormality is the indication for pregnancy interruption. This finding is in accord with the previously discussed rubella data, which similarly dealt with (potential) fetal abnormality as the indication for abortion.

Psychological trauma is implicit in the loss of a desired pregnancy; thus the reaction to selective abortion is closely akin to the grief response to perinatal death. In contrast, elective abortion (on demand) usually involves the termination of an unwanted pregnancy and is therefore as likely to produce relief as regret.

Selective abortion, however, is more than the passive loss of an emotionally invested pregnancy. The parents, in accepting direct responsibility for the painful decision to abort, must assume an active and 'causative' role in their pregnancy loss. The conflict imposed upon the parents by the discovery of a fetal defect may be conceptualized as follows:

	P		
Socially acceptable prevention of birth of defective child	A R	Desire for child	Continuation
←———————	E	– – – – – →	of
– – – – – →	N	← —————	pregnancy
Personal anti-abortion attitudes (moral, religious)	T	Anticipated burden of bearing defective child	
	S		

The wish to avoid the anticipated burden of bearing a defective child usually supersedes the desire for a child and may lead a couple to interrupt pregnancy even in the face of preexistent moral or religious objections to abortion. Frequently, depression is the price of this internal psychic transaction.

As already implied, the timing of selective abortion in relation to quickening may contribute to the psychological trauma of the procedure. In the instance of elective abortion (on demand), second trimester procedures often are associated with negative psychiatric sequelae (Brewer, 1978). However, a delay in seeking elective abortion often reflects an ambivalence toward pregnancy that is not shared by women who postpone an abortion decision due to the practical demands of prenatal diagnosis. It may be difficult for parents to avoid thinking of the fetus as a baby by 20 weeks of pregnancy. Parents often prefer to maintain an abstract rather than a concrete notion of the fetus' identity; in order to serve this need, the gender of an abnormal fetus should be divulged to the parents only if specifically requested and after serious consideration of this issue.

The actual medical procedure employed for second trimester induced abortion also may contribute to the emotional trauma of the experience (Kaltreider et al., 1979). The vaginal 'delivery' of a non-viable fetus following prostaglandin administration (or similar techniques) has been especially traumatic for selective abortion recipients. The stark reality of the observed fetus denies the opportunity to consider the abortion in abstract and more comfortable terms. In contrast, dilatation and evacuation (D & E) under general anaesthesia circumvents the physical discomforts of labour and the emotional discomfort of a direct confrontation with the fetus. However, ultimate resolution of the grief process actually may be facilitated by the direct contact with the fetus that is necessitated by a prostaglandin abortion. Being forced to face the fetus, the parents are required to acknowledge and deal with their grief. If the parents are inclined to inspect the fetus, it is helpful if the counsellor or a medical representative is available to modulate the emotional intensity of this encounter. It is important to point out any subtle fetal anomalies that might confirm the prenatal diagnosis and help the parents to justify their decision to end the pregnancy. At the same time parents' injured self-esteem could benefit from attention directed to the normal features of the fetus.

Further contributing to the emotional burden of selective abortion is the sense of guilt associated with genetic disease. The parents not only have failed in their attempt to reproduce in a child their favourable qualities, but added to this sense of failure is a recognition that their own undesirable attributes (advanced age or carrier status) have been responsible for the fetal abnormality. Guilt feelings may be particularly damaging when genetic responsibility is perceived to derive from only one parent (Blumberg, 1974). Thus, in the case of X-linked disorders, the mother may be blamed or blame herself for the condition occurring within her family. Carrier status is much less stigmatizing in autosomal recessive conditions; in such disorders, parents may share a sense of genetic responsibility and view their misfortune as a vagary of random mating. In rare instances, one parent may suffer from an autosomal dominant disease, which, when diagnosed in the fetus, leads to the decision to terminate a pregnancy. This course of action may be regarded as a denial of self-worth as well as a reflection of guilt feelings associated with the transmission of a genetic disease.

In families with a prior history of genetic disease, selective abortion may rekindle the negative emotions associated with the previous birth of an affected child. In addition, the implications of prenatal diagnosis extend to the future. The diagnosis of a fetal defect leads to an inescapable awareness that a similar outcome is possible in any subsequent pregnancies. For this reason, some couples elect sterilization following selective abortion. To whatever extent possible, the counsellor should discourage any such permanent decisions until the parents have recovered from the turbulence of the abortion experience. For some families, the desire for a child is strong enough to justify further reproductive efforts despite the trauma of selective abortion. Other families express their ambivalence by deferring further reproductive decisions indefinitely (Blumberg, 1974; Blumberg et al., 1975).

The negative psychological sequelae of selective abortion may be quite persistent; resolution of emotional problems requires the application of the couple's individual and joint adaptive resources. Not infrequently, the subsequent birth of a healthy child serves as the catalyst for emotional recovery by restoring previously diminished self-esteem and by satisfying the goal of successful reproduction. For families unwilling to risk further pregnancies, adoption may offer the oportunity to experience parental fulfilment. Relatively few families have experienced the misfortune of abnormal prenatal diagnostic results in successive pregnancies. However, when it occurs, this dual tragedy may be followed by chronic depression and an unwillingness to risk further pregnancies. Similar consequences may ensue when a fetal defect is encountered by a family with a previous history of an abnormal liveborn.

The emotional trauma inherent in prenatal diagnosis occasionally has been invoked as an argument against the procedure, but this argument fails to consider prenatal diagnosis in the context of its alternatives. It is not surprising that women who have received normal amniocentesis results would almost unanimously elect to undergo this procedure again in subsequent pregnancies and would recommend prenatal diagnosis to others (Golbus et al., 1974; Finley et al., 1977). More significantly, most couples who have experienced the turmoil associated with an abnormal result and selective abortion also would resort to amniocentesis again in future pregnancies (Blumberg et al., 1975). This behaviour can be comprehended only by recognizing that the alternatives to prenatal diagnosis are associated with their own emotional burdens. A decision to forego further reproduction would entail a frustration of the desire to reproduce and could deprive the family of the much wanted normal child. A decision to undertake a new pregnancy without the benefit of prenatal diagnosis would expose the family to the risk of bearing another defective child and to the anxieties attendant to this risk. Therefore, for most families, the option of prenatal diagnosis is pursued despite their intimate understanding of the potential emotional implications of this course of action.

Prenatal diagnostic counselling

Since psychological disturbance is a normal rather than a pathological response to prenatal diagnosis, counselling efforts should support the family's attempts to cope with the emotional stress accompanying the procedure. Because prenatal diagnosis can exert its influence even prior to conception, the first goal of the care provider should be the dissemination of genetic knowledge to the public. Informed procreative decisions require a prior awareness of reproductive risk and of the methods available (or unavailable) to deal with this risk.

Once having embarked upon a pregnancy, the couple considering prenatal diagnosis should receive prediagnostic counselling at the earliest opportunity. Beyond the information transfer required for an educated decision, attention should be directed to the emotional issues of prenatal diagnosis. Supportive counselling is especially valuable to families at high genetic risk and to those with previous negative reproductive experiences. The specific counselling strategy employed (e.g. group, individual, videotape assisted, etc.) is less important than the predication of counselling upon a sensitivity to the individual emotional needs of the pregnant couple.

Prediagnostic counselling must explain the pertinent procedures, their risks, and their limitations. Conveying this information often diminishes the fears of maternal pain or injury and of the unknown aspects of the procedure (Matthews and Henry, 1979). Unfortunately, preexisting fears of fetal loss or injury may be magnified by the counsellor's required enumeration of these risks.

Counselling should also include a consideration of the consequences of an abnormal result. Discussion of this issue is likely to increase concerns related to the possibility of abortion (Matthews and Henry, 1979). However, individuals who successfully resolve their ambivalence toward selective abortion (and are firm in their intention to terminate pregnancy in the event that a fetal anomaly is discovered) may experience a subsequent reduction in their level of anxiety (Beeson and Golbus, 1979).

Although it is well known that the waiting period between the performance of amniocentesis and the communication of its result is a stressful phase of diagnosis, there have been few attempts to provide emotional support during this interval. Some centres do contact families during the waiting period in order to provide assurance that a cell culture has been established. There is some evidence that this contact is effective in allaying the concerns of couples with high levels of anxiety (Beeson and Golbus, 1979).

In most instances, the communication of a normal test result is the final contact with the pregnant couple (excluding follow-up medical data collected at or after the time of delivery). However, the continuing concern expressed by some women, even after a normal amniocentesis result (Robinson et al., 1975), emphasizes the need for a more thorough assessment of the psychological elements of later pregnancy following prenatal diagnosis.

The enormous emotional impact of an abnormal test result requires immediate crisis counselling in order to promote an optimal decision within the temporal constraints imposed by medicolegal considerations. Parents, of course, must first understand the clinical implications of the detected abnormality. Realistic alternatives must be presented in a non-coercive manner. When the two parents disagree about the course of action to be taken, the use of threat and innuendo by one partner may produce long standing remorse and jeopardize marital stability. Recognizing these factors, the counsellor should attempt to facilitate a decision that can be accepted by both parents. However, with such high stakes, it may be impossible for individuals to agree upon a mutually acceptable course of action. In this instance, dissolution of the parental relationship often is the unfortunate result.

A decision to continue pregnancy after the discovery of a fetal defect requires supportive counselling that should extend throughout pregnancy and beyond the birth of the affected child. If abortion is elected, a detailed description of the planned procedure must be presented. Post-abortional supportive counselling frequently is indicated. The provision of post-abortional results (i.e. pathological, biochemical, or cytogenetic) confirming the presence of the predicted fetal defect may help the family to rationalize their decision to terminate the pregnancy. At this time, the counsellor should begin to assess the influence of the diagnostic experience upon future reproductive attitudes. Contraceptive advice may be appropriate in some cases. It should not be forgotten that other family members may also require supportive counselling following selective abortion. Older siblings of the aborted fetus, especially if they are afflicted with the same condition discovered in the fetus, may experience a consequent devaluation of self-esteem. Only by openly addressing the emotional needs of all involved in the diagnostic experience (perhaps including medical personnel) can one hope to minimize the psychological trauma of selective abortion.

Summary

In the future, prenatal diagnosis will be employed by a growing number of families as technology expands diagnostic capabilities. For some couples, the availability of prenatal diagnosis will be the critical factor in their decision to undertake pregnancy and confront their genetic risks. For others, prenatal diagnosis will offer the opportunity to reduce the normal anxieties of the second half of pregnancy. For a few, prenatal diagnosis may precipitate an emotional crisis by revealing a fetal abnormality. Significant psychological trauma may be an unavoidable consequence of selective abortion, but the alternative birth of a defective child is usually accompanied by even more intense feelings of guilt and depression. The necessity of psychological counselling during the prenatal diagnostic process is apparent. Equally obvious is the need for further scientific research into the emotionl facets of fetal genetic assessment. Only by acknowledging and further exploring these important issues will prenatal diagnosticians realize their full potential to serve the psychological and physical needs of an informed reproductive populace.

References

Adler, B. and Kushnick, T. (1982). Genetic counseling in prenatally diagnosed trisomy 18 and 21: psychosocial aspects. *Pediatrics* **69**, 94–99.

Ashery, R. S. (1981). Communication openness with friends, relatives, and children of couples having amniocentesis. *Prenatal Diagnosis* **1**, 153–156.

Astbury, J. and Walters, W. A. W. (1979). Amniocentesis in the early second trimester of pregnancy and maternal anxiety. *Aust. Fam. Physician* **8**, 595–599.

Beeson, D. and Golbus, M. S. (1979). Anxiety engendered by amniocentesis. *Birth Defects* **15**, 191–197.

Bibring, G., Dwyer, T., Huntington, D. and Valenstein, A. (1961). A study of the psychological processes in pregnancy and the earliest mother–child relationship. *Psychoanal. Study Child* **16**, 9–24.

Bibring, G. and Valenstein, A. (1976). Psychological aspects of pregnancy. *Clin. Obstet. Gynecol.* **19**, 357–371.

Blumberg, B. (1974). 'Psychic Sequelae of Selective Abortion'. Yale University MD thesis, New Haven, Connecticut.

Blumberg, B. and Golbus, M. (1975). Psychological sequelae of elective abortion. *West. J. Med.* **123**, 188–193.

Blumberg, B. Golbus, M. and Hanson, K. (1975). The psychological sequelae of abortion performed for a genetic indication. *Am. J. Obstet. Gynecol.* **122**, 799–808.

Brewer, C. (1978). Induced abortion after feeling fetal movements: its causes and emotional consequences. *J. Biosoc. Sci.* **10**, 203–208.

Burton, B. K., Dillard, R. G. and Clark, E. N. (1982). Anxiety associated with maternal serum alpha-fetoprotein (AFP) screening. *Am. J. Hum. Genet.* **34**, 83A.

Chervin, A., Farnsworth, P. B., Freedman, W. L., Duncan, P. A. and Shapiro, L. R. (1977). Amniocentesis for prenatal diagnosis – subjective patient response. *N.Y. State J. Med.* **77**, 1406–1408.

Donnai, P., Charles, N. and Harris, R. (1981). Attitudes of patients after 'genetic' termination of pregnancy. *Br. Med. J.* **282**, 621–622.

Dixson, B., Richards, T. L., Reinsch, S., Edrich, V. B., Matson, M. R. and Jones, O. W. (1981). Midtrimester amniocentesis – subjective maternal responses. *J. Reprod. Med.* **26**, 10–16.

Fava, G. A., Kellner, R., Michelacci, L., Trombini, G., Pathak, D., Orlandi, C. and Bovicelli, L. (1982). Psychological reactions to amniocentesis: a controlled study. *Am. J. Obstet. Gynecol.* **143**, 509–513.

Fearn, J., Hibbard, B. M., Laurence, K. M., Roberts, A. and Robinson, J. O. (1982). Screening for neural-tube defects and maternal anxiety. *Br. J. Obstet. Gynaecol.* **89**, 218–221.

Finley, S., Varner, P., Vinson, P. and Finley, W. (1977). Participants' reaction to amniocentesis and prenatal genetic studies. *J.A.M.A.* **238**, 2377–2379.

Fletcher, J. (1972). The brink: the parent–child bond in the genetic revolution. *Theological Studies* **33**, 457–485.

Golbus, M., Conte, F., Schneider, E. and Epstein, C. (1974). Intrauterine diagnosis of genetic defects: results, problems and follow-up of one hundred cases in a prenatal genetic detection center. *Am. J. Obstet. Gynecol.* **118**, 897–905.

Hook, E. and Wiley, A (1979). Suppose amniocentesis were not available? Results of a survey. *Am. J. Hum. Genet.* **31**, 12A.

Hsia, Y., Leung, F. and Carter, L. (1979). Attitudes toward amniocentesis: Surveys of families with spina bifida children. In 'Service and Education in Medical Genetics' (I. Porter and E. Hook, Eds). Academic Press, New York and London.

Kaltreider, N., Goldsmith, S. and Margolis, A. (1979). The impact of midtrimester abortion techniques on patients and staff. *Am. J. Obstet. Gynecol.* **135**, 235–238.

Laurence, K. M. and Morris, J. (1981). The effect of the introduction of prenatal diagnosis on the reproductive history of women at increased risk from neural tube defects. *Prenatal Diagnosis* **1**, 51–60.

Matthews, A. and Henry, G. (1979). Learning, satisfaction, and anxiety parameters in a preamniocentesis genetic counseling program: A comparison of genetic counselors and a videotaped program. *Am. J. Hum. Genet.* **31**, 124A.

Milne, L. S. and Rich, O. J. (1981). Cognitive and affective aspects of the responses of pregnant women to sonography. *Matern. Child Nurs. J.* **10**, 15–39.

Morris, D. (1976). Parental reactions to perinatal death. *Proc. R. Soc. Med.* **69**, 837–838.

Myrianthopoulos, N. and Aronson, S. (1966). Population dynamics of Tay-Sachs disease. I. Reproductive fitness and selection. *Am. J. Hum. Genet.* **18**, 313–327.

Robinson, J., Tennes, K. and Robinson, A. (1975). Amniocentesis: its impact on mothers and infants. A 1-year follow-up study. *Clin. Genet.* **8**, 97–106.

Silvestre, D. and Fresco, N. (1980). Reactions to prenatal diagnosis: an analysis of 87 interviews. *Am. J. Orthopsychiatr.* **50**, 610–617.

Simon, N., Senturia, A. and Rothman, D. (1967). Psychiatric illness following therapeutic abortion. *Am. J. Psychiatr.* **124**, 59–65.

Simon, N., Rothman, D., Goff, J. and Senturia, A. (1969). Psychological factors related to spontaneous and therapeutic abortion. *Am. J. Obstet. Gynecol.* **104**, 799–808.

Solnit, A. and Stark, M. (1961). Mourning and the birth of a defective child. *Psychoanal. Study Child.* **16**, 523–537.

Verjaal, M., Leschot, N. J. and Treffers, P. E. (1982). Women's experiences with second trimester prenatal diagnosis. *Prenatal Diagnosis* **2**, 195–209.

14 *Training in Genetic Counselling*

PETER MAGUIRE

Introduction

If a doctor is to provide genetic counselling effectively several tasks must be fulfilled. He must interview in a way which encourages the patient to disclose all relevant data, otherwise, his diagnosis may be inaccurate and the mechanism of inheritance poorly understood. He has to cover sensitive areas such as the incidence and nature of any stillbirths or miscarriages without alienating the patient or imputing blame for hereditary disease.

Once the diagnosis has been established and the genetic risks determined the doctor faces the problem of how to convey this information to the patient so that it is fully understood but without alarming the patient unnecessarily. Hearing such news may upset some people or they may find it hard to accept. It is, therefore, important that the doctor allows time for the news to be absorbed and then checks whether it has been understood correctly. Unless this is done routinely the person being counselled may harbour serious misconceptions and make an inappropriate decision. If they are upset by the information given they are especially likely to misinterpret it. The doctor should check how the patient feels about what has been said and clarify the reasons for any upset. If he omits this his attempts at reassurance are likely to be inappropriate to the patient's needs and concerns.

Once he is sure that the diagnosis and its implications have been grasped the doctor has to help the patient clarify the possible options and their likely consequences so an informed decision can then be made. However well the patient has been counselled there may still be doubts and misunderstandings and uncertainty about what decision to make or how to handle the future. The patient should, therefore, be encouraged to feel that he or she can contact the doctor at any any time to ask further questions or discuss particular aspects. Such further contact will also enable the doctor to monitor how well

Psychological Aspects Genetic Counselling

the patient has been coping with the situation and determine if any problems have arisen.

These tasks can only be performed properly if those carrying out genetic counselling possess the relevant skills. While it has been widely assumed that most doctors acquire these skills during their medical training this assumption has been seriously challenged by studies which have directly observed doctor–patient interactions. They have found a consistent pattern of deficiencies irrespective of the type of doctors studied or their length of experience (Maguire, 1981).

Deficiencies in key skills

Deficiencies in counselling skills have been observed and studied in both hospital doctors and family doctors (general practitioners).

Hospital doctors

Weiner and Nathanson (1976) observed short interviews between 145 doctors in higher medical training and medical patients. They found that the patients were rarely allowed to tell their stories in their own way. Instead, they were asked too many questions and little attempt was made to clarify or understand their complaints. When the patients asked questions about their condition these were answered only rarely. Similar deficiencies were noted by Platt and McMath (1979) who watched 300 interviews conducted by a group of physicians who represented the whole spectrum of clinical experience. They concluded that there were certain main defects in their skills.

Their interviews showed a 'low therapeutic contact'. They explained little about the purpose of what they were doing and were not very supportive or understanding in the comments they made. They did not usually ask how patients were feeling about their condition and were poor at giving reassurance. While many patients gave the doctor's verbal cues about their key concerns these were commonly missed or ignored. Platt and McMath also considered that the data obtained were inadequate ('flawed data base') since the physicians failed to check if the patients had any important problems other than their presenting complaints, and did not ask about their daily lives or possibility of concurrent stresses. While some patients were difficult to interview or appeared upset few doctors appeared to pause to consider what the reasons might be ('failure to generate hypotheses'). Consequently, they got into difficulties which could have been avoided. Since the doctors were working in hospital they were hearing the patients' stories second hand. They had already mentioned their complaints at least once to the referring doctor. Despite this, the physicians took these accounts on trust and few bothered to find out for themselves exactly what the patient had experienced when they suffered symptoms like 'chest pain' or 'depression' ('failure to demand Primary Data'). Overall, the physicians showed a 'high control style'. They tolerated silences poorly, did too much of the talking, asked questions in a form which suggested an answer and were too quick in deciding what was the main problem. Once they had pinpointed what seemed to be the main problem they did not screen for the possibility of any others.

Another important theme running through these studies was the reluctance of physicians to cover psychological and social aspects of illness and this was confirmed by Aloia and Jones (1976). Few patients were asked about their home or family life or about how the illness had affected them. Duffy *et al.* (1980) similarly found that psychosocial aspects were neglected. 73 per cent of the doctors they studied who were working in medical outpatients failed to establish what was their patients' understanding of their illness and only 35 per cent asked how they had been affected emotionally.

Doctors working in other specialties show similar deficiencies. For example, surgeons appear very directive and reluctant to deal with any aspect other than the obvious presenting physical problem. They ignore important verbal and non-verbal cues about patients' concerns and reactions to illness. Their reassurance is often ineffective because they have not first established what patients are worried about (Maguire, 1976). Only rarely do they establish what the patients think and feel about their illness. Contrary to what might have been expected, psychiatrists have also been found to have difficulty establishing a productive relationship, listening properly and handling emotionally loaded material (Junek *et al.*, 1979). They are more likely to miss physical problems because of their preoccupation with mental illness and patients' beliefs that psychiatrists do not deal with physical matters.

Paediatricians have to deal with young children and might, therefore, have developed considerable skills in communication. If so, this was not apparent in a study of interactions within a paediatric clinic (Korsch *et al.*, 1968). The paediatricians wasted much time through not identifying the mothers' concerns and expectations. They dealt poorly with questions and missed or ignored key cues. Little attempt was made to reassure mothers who felt in some way responsible for their child's illness and what attempts were made were usually unsuccessful. Consequently, only 24 per cent of mothers had revealed their true concerns about their child by the time they had left the clinic.

General practitioners

General practitioners who are called upon to counsel have the potential advantage of knowing the patient already and usually being the first to hear about a problem. However, they have also often been found to be lacking in the skills relevant to genetic counselling.

When Byrne and Long (1976) recorded over 2000 consultations on audiotape they found a considerable number of problems which were similar to those found in hospital doctors. The general practitioners tended to follow a set sequence of questions which was little affected by what the patients said or what their expectations and concerns were. They seemed too eager to seize on the first problem offered and assume that it was the only one. When patients tried to discuss their feelings the practitioners attempted to stifle such expression and keep the consultation at a superficial level. This suggested that they were trying to avoid getting close to their patients and this was borne out by other observations. They were reluctant to clarify what patients had really experienced or cover psychological and social aspects. Patients were usually given little opportunity to ask questions and the reassurance offered by the doctors was often premature and inappropriate. Nor was much effort taken to establish patients' own perceptions and attitudes. Often the practitioners seemed to have some preconception about what would be wrong with the patient, even though this was often wrong. Instead of assisting them, their prior knowledge of the patient often led them to prejudge the issue and make an inaccurate diagnosis.

Verby *et al.* (1979) confirmed these findings in a small sample of general practitioners and found that they were not remedied by experience. Practitioners themselves have acknowledged these difficulties (Bennett *et al.*, 1978) and admitted that they find it especially hard to convey that a problem is trivial or break bad news.

Given the nature and scale of the deficiencies in skills found in both hospital doctors and general practitioners it seems unlikely that many possess the skills relevant to genetic counselling. The reasons for this will now be considered since they affect decisions about training for genetic counselling.

Gaps in medical training

Training in the relevant skills is usually limited to how to take a history. Few doctors have been given any explicit or formal guidance about how to convey information to patients, break bad news, provide reassurance and talk with relatives. Even training in history-taking as generally conducted suffers from serious limitations.

Guidance is usually limited to telling students via handouts or lectures what questions they should ask so that they cover all possible physical symptoms and signs. Little attention is devoted to psychological or social aspects. For example, the social history often covers only cigarette and alcohol consumption. Nor do guidelines usually include how to begin or end the interview, keep patients to the point, respond to and clarify verbal and non-verbal cues, reassure patients, ask questions, obtain precise information or avoid unnecessary repetition. Instead it is generally believed that doctors will acquire these skills by watching their teachers at work with patients and relatives.

Yet, few if any of these teachers will have been trained adequately in these skills. Consequently, doctors in training will be modelling themselves on teachers who are likely to be deficient in at least some of the relevant skills. Unfortunately there is little chance of the trainee or 'expert' realizing this. For the level of a doctor's skills in communicating with patients is commonly judged on the basis of his written histories when he reports these to the teacher. The doctor is not actually observed while interviewing and so, deficiencies will go unnoticed especially as there is little relationship between how he interviewed and his written history. The teacher may continue to believe that his teaching is effective and his trainees are proficient. Both undergraduate and postgraduate training rely on this apprenticeship method. So it is not surprising that deficiencies are not remedied and may become more marked (Verby et al., 1980).

The avoidance of difficult issues, like emotionally loaded topics and breaking bad news, by many doctors is easy to understand when it is accepted that they are given so little help during their training in the learning of key skills.

Training for genetic counselling

Training must begin with the realization that the potential counsellor may, through no fault of his own, lack some of the key skills or may not be confident in applying them. The first step, therefore, is to make the skills explicit.

Providing a model

For each of the tasks involved in genetic counselling the areas to be covered and the techniques to be used should be made explicit. They should be detailed in a handout and, where possible, demonstrated in action by an expert using audio or videotape recordings. Since there appear to be few if any commercially available demonstration tapes these may have to be made by the teacher himself.

The comments on obtaining a history should include a description of general techniques (Maguire and Rutter, 1976). They should pay particular attention to the need for good eye contact, precision of data and ability to recognize and clarify verbal and non-verbal cues. For example, when explaining that she wants advice about the wisdom of having another baby the mother of a mentally handicapped child may look upset. Saying 'You seem upset, would you like to tell me what's bothering you?' encourages her to disclose that she is terrified of having a second handicapped child because she is only barely managing to look after the first one. She even doubts her capacity to cope if the child is healthy. Such upset and feelings of failure as a parent and frustration at not having a normal child to love, are commonly present and the patient should be helped to express them if any cues are given.

In trying to explain why they themselves or a relative have or are at risk of developing a given disease they search for tangible reasons such as a bad fall or exposure to radiation in pregnancy or think some other relative had a similar illness. It is most important that whenever possible such claims are verified. Otherwise the doctor may be misled into seeing a connection between events which did not really exist and fall into this trap of searching too eagerly for a meaning. Given the delicate nature of such probing for possible hereditary mechanisms the doctor must be alert to the possibility that his questions may upset or alarm the patient. He must avoid implying someone was to blame but be aware that the patient might do this. The doctor must do his utmost to avoid false attribution of responsibility and encourage open discussion of any feelings of anger and resentment.

When conveying the diagnosis and future risk the doctor has an unenviable task if his news is bad. However, he should do so in private and begin by explaining that he is now going to explain the risks of whatever situation he has been consulted about and break the news honestly but gently. Thus, he might begin by saying to a woman who wants to know the chances of her son contracting a muscle disease 'let me try and explain his chances since that's what you came to see me for. There is a 50 per cent chance he could be alright'. He should then pause, allow the mother time to absorb the information and ask 'how are you feeling about what I have just said?' She might say 'I just don't believe you' so suggesting that she is finding it too painful to accept. Alternatively and more likely she may say 'That's awful, that's what I've always feared'. The doctor should then clarify why she feels upset or angry and encourage her to express these feelings. This usually lessens the intensity of the feelings and makes them more manageable. He should then ask if she has any further questions. In this way he goes at the mother's pace and avoids making guesses about how much she should or should not be told. If further questions are asked these should be answered honestly but the hopeful aspects emphasised. Thus, he will emphasize the 50 per cent chance of the son staying well rather than the converse.

In discussing possible scenarios when requested to do so by the patient, the doctor must avoid false optimism or reassurance, for the patient who asks to be put fully in the picture is likely to cope much better if he or she has a realistic grasp of the possibilities. Similarly, a patient who replies to the doctor's enquiry that she does not wish to ask any questions or learn any more should be heeded.

When the request for counselling has come from a person with a partner it is important that he or she is given the opportunity to be seen with the partner if they so wish. While such openness between a couple can be painful for them because they wish to protect each other it allows them to give support and discuss critical decisions.

Deciding to withold the true risk despite a patient's request for the truth is unhelpful and often provokes enormous bitterness and resentment when the patient realizes he or she was not trusted with the truth. When the future is uncertain some patients may request 'markers' that is, indicators of whether the feared condition is developing so that they can do something constructive about it. These requests should be met since most people cope best with uncertainty in that way.

If the doctor has been empathic throughout, that is, he has given the person who sought help the feeling that he does understand the predicament she faces and her feelings, it is likely she will continue to use him as a source of advice and support. Before discussing such future contact it is helpful if the doctor checks if she is happy with what has been discussed and has all the information she needs. If the discussion has concerned a common problem like fibrocystic disease or Down's syndrome the doctor can ask if she might find it helpful to talk with a mother who faced the same predicament. However, to suggest to a person who is likely to have a hereditary disease that 'there are lots of people like you' is likely to cause upset unless he or she has had a full opportunity to discuss their own worries and feelings first.

Practice

In order to determine how well a doctor counsels and what he needs to improve his counselling, he should be given a precise task and asked to practise under controlled conditions. Thus, he could be asked to concentrate on taking a history in order to establish a diagnosis and produce an estimate of risk. He could practise giving information, breaking bad news or clarifying possible options. He should be allowed a finite amount of time and told that it is up to him to end within that limit. This allows the issue of whether he makes best use of his time to be discussed.

Feedback

It has been found that skills are much more likely to be acquired if training includes the recording of performance on audiotape or videotape followed by feedback with a tutor (Maguire *et al.*, 1978). Audiotape recording is the easiest to use and allows most of the relevant skills to be rated. Vidoetape recording has the advantage that non-verbal behaviours can be shown and discussed but technical assistance, and a specially equipped room, are necessary.

Recording of a counselling session is acceptable to most patients provided the doctor explains that it is to help him look at what he is doing rather than focus on them. However, it is easier to look at the component tasks individually by asking the doctor to interview a simulated patient. Such simulators are best trained by asking them to play the part of a patient who came for genetic counselling. They are given a clear case history and asked to alter it so that it feels congruent with their own biography. They may then be interviewed, to see if they can sustain the role, and given video feedback about their performance (Maguire *et al.*, 1977). They may be drawn from existing hospital staff or obtained by advertising in the local newspaper. While doubts have been expressed about simulated patients it has been established that the way doctors interview such patients matches closely how they relate to real patients (Sanson-Fisher and Poole, 1980).

Tasks

Whether real or simulated patients are used they should cover the range of problems found within the field of genetic counselling. This might include: a mother who is deciding if she should risk having a child; a pregnant woman worried about the kind of baby she is likely to have; a woman who has recently given birth to a child suffering from a hereditary disease; a couple who want to adopt a child but are worried about an adverse history; a couple asking for advice about sterilization; and a young man who is afraid he will develop a hereditary disease which only declares itself in later life.

Teaching

The teacher must understand the skills being taught and have some means of evaluating performance. Otherwise, he will not be able to identify strengths and and weaknesses systematically. Global or analogue scales which require the teacher to indicate how well or badly a doctor used a required technique such as 'responding to verbal cues' are probably the most useful (Maguire *et al.*, 1978).

This feedback teaching is as effective when given within small groups providing the teacher observes certain rules. He should focus both on the data to be covered and the skills which are to be used. Strengths should be highlighted before weaknesses are exposed and the 'hot seat' approach should be avoided where one doctor is criticised by the remainder. The doctors should also be encouraged to say how they felt about being observed and the task that they were given. The willingness to practise three or four times and receive feedback should result in considerable learning for most doctors. However, there will be a few who fail to learn. They might respond to training which focuses on the areas they find most difficult and includes feedback from the patient about what it was like to be counselled in that way. The use of a third person who asks the doctor and patient to discuss step by step how the session went has also been advocated (Kagan *et al.*, 1969).

Training the tutors

A key question is who should carry out this training and how should they be trained? A recent study has suggested that a doctor, psychologist or nurse can do it effectively provided they have watched demonstration tapes and are clear about the principles to be followed and the skills that are to be taught (Fairbairn *et al.*, 1983). What is not clear is whether or not they should have first been trained in counselling skills in exactly the same way as the doctors they are going to teach.

Evolving the methods

The methods of counselling discussed so far have appeared acceptable and effective when carried out in clinical practice (Maguire *et al.*, 1980). In the specific area of genetic counselling some skills might prove to be of more value than others. This will only become clear if vigorous attempts are made to link the use of specified skills to both short and longer term outcomes in those counselled, particularly the patients' psychological and social adjustment. The training methods can then be modified to take account of such findings.

Conclusions

Genetic counselling requires that the doctor possess certain key skills. Unfortunately, he is not as likely to have acquired them as he might think.

This is due to serious deficiencies in current medical training. Only the adoption of systematic observation and feedback of performance is likely to affect favourably the acquisition of the relevant skills and ensure the provision of effective counsellors.

References

Aloia, J. F. and Jonas, E. (1976). Skills in history-taking and physical examination. *J. Med. Educ.* **51**, 410–415.

Bennet, A., Knox, J. D. E. and Morrison, A. T. (1978). Difficulties in consultations reported by doctors in general practice. *J. Royal Coll. G.P.* **28**, 646–651.

Byrne, P. S. and Long, B. E. L. (1976). 'Doctors talking to patients'. HMSO, London.

Duffy, D. L., Hammerman, L. and Cohen, A. (1980). Communication skills of house officers. A study in a medical clinic. *Ann. Int. Med.* **93**, 354–357.

Fairbairn, S., Maguire, P. and Sanson-Fisher, R. W. (1983). Expert versus novice teaching in interviewing training. *J. Med. Educ.* (in press).

Junek, W., Burra, P. and Leichner, P. (1979). Teaching interviewing skills by encountering patients. *J. Med. Educ.* **54**, 402–407.

Kagan, N., Schauble, P., Reznikoff, A., Danish, S. J. and Krathwohl, D. R. (1969). Interpersonal process recall. *J. Nerv. Ment. Dis.* **148**, 365–374.

Korsch, B. M., Grozzi, E. K. and Francis, V. (1968). Gaps in doctor–patient communication. 1. Doctor–patient interaction and patient satisfaction. *Pediatrics* **42**, 855–871.

Maguire, G. P., Clarke, D. and Jolly, B. (1977). An experimental comparison of three courses in history-taking skills for medical students. *Med. Educ.* **11**, 175–182.

Maguire, P. and Argyle, P. P. (1981). Doctor–patient skills. *In* 'Social skills and health' (P. Maguire, Ed.), pp. 55–81. Methuen, London.

Maguire, P. (1976). The psychological and social sequelae of mastectomy. *In* 'Modern perspectives in the psychiatric aspects of surgery' (J. G. Howells, Ed.), pp. 390–420. Brunner Mazel, New York.

Maguire, P. and Rutter, D. (1976). The development and evaluation of an interviewing model and training procedure. *In* 'Communication between doctors and patients' (A. E. Bennett, Ed.), pp. 45–74. Oxford University Press, London.

Maguire, P., Roe, P., Goldberg, D., Jones, S., Hyde, C. and O'Dowd, T. (1980). The value of feedback in teaching interview skills to medical students. *Psychol. Med.* **8**, 695–704.

Maguire, P., Tait, A., Brooke, M., Thomas, C. and Sellwood, R. (1980). Effect of counselling on the psychiatric morbidity associated with mastectomy. *Brit. Med. J.* **281**, 1454–1456.

Platt, F. W. and McMath, J. C. (1979). Clinical hypocompetence. The Interview. *Ann. Int. Med.* **91**, 898–902.

Sanson-Fisher, R. W. and Poole, A. D. (1980). Simulated patients and the assessment of medical students' interpersonal skills. *Med. Educ.* **14**, 249–253.

Verby, J. E., Holden, P. and Davis, R. H. (1979). Peer review of consultations in primary care: the use of audiovisual recordings. *Brit. Med. J.* **1**, 1686–1688.

Verby, J. E., Davis, R. H. and Holden, P. (1980). A study of the interviewing skills of trainee assistants in general practice. *Patient Coun. Hlth. Educ.* **2**, 68–71.

Weissman, M. M. and Klerman, G. L. (1977). The chronic depressive in the community: unrecognised and poorly treated. *Comp. Psychiat.* **18**, 523–531.

Appendix

Table A1   Risks (%) to offspring in unifactorial disorders

	Progeny of affected male		Progeny of heterozygous female	
Mode of inheritance	Normal	Affected	Normal	Affected
Male progeny				
Autosomal recessive	100	0	100	0
Autosomal dominant	50	50	50	50
Autosomal dominant (male limited)	50	50	50	50
X-linked recessive	100	0	50	50
X-linked dominant	100	0	50	50
Female progeny				
Autosomal recessive	100	0	100	0
Autosomal dominant	50	50	50	50
Autosomal dominant (male limited)	50	50(c)	50	50(c)
X-linked recessive	0	100(c)	50	50(c)
X-linked dominant	0	100	50	50

(c) indicates a carrier, usually unaffected

Table A.2   Risks at birth of Down's syndrome due to trisomy 21 in relation to maternal age

Maternal age	Risks
20	1 in 2000
25	1 in 1200
30	1 in 800
35	1 in 400
40	1 in 100
45	1 in 30

Table A.3 Risks (%) of Down's syndrome when one of the parents carries a translocation (C = carrier; N = normal)

Translocation	Father	Mother	Risks
13–15/21	N	C	10–15
	C	N	5
21/22	N	C	10–15
	C	N	5
21/21	C	N	100
	N	C	100

(NB occasionally a translocation only occurs in the affected child and neither parent when the risk of recurrence is about 1%)

Table A.4 Empiric risks (%) for some common disorders (from Emery, A. E. H. (1983) 'Elements of Medical Genetics' 6th edition. Churchill-Livingstone, Edinburgh and London, with permission)

Disorder	Incidence	Sex ratio M:F	Normal parents having a second affected child	Affected parent having an affected child	Affected parent having a second affected child
Anencephaly	0·20	1:2	5[a]	—	—
Asthma	3–4	1:1	10	26	—
Cerebral palsy	0·20	3:2	1[c]	—	—
Cleft palate only	0·04	2:3	2	7	15
Cleft lip ± cleft palate	0·10	3:2	4	4	10
Club foot	0·10	2:1	3	3	10

Congenital heart disease (all types)	0·50	1:1	1–4	1–4	10
Diabetes mellitus (juvenile, insulin-dependent)	0·20	1:1	6	1–2	—
Dislocation of hip	0·07	1:6	6	12	36
Exomphalos (omphalocoele)	0·02	1:1	<1	—	—
Epilepsy ('idiopathic')	0·50	1:1	5	5	10
Hirschsprung's disease					
short segment	0·02	4:1	3	2	—
long segment			12	—	—
Hydrocephalus (isolated, not XR)	0·05	1:1	3[b]	—	—
Hypospadias (in males)	0·20	—	10	10	—
Manic-depressive psychosis	0·40	2:3	10–15	10–15	—
Mental retardation ('idiopathic')	0·30–0·50	1:1	3–5	10	20
Profound childhood deafness	0·10	1:1	10	8	—
Pyloric stenosis	0·30	5:1			
male index			2	4	13
female index			10	17	38
Renal agenesis (bilat.)	0·01	3:1			
male index			3	—	—
female index			7	—	—
Schizophrenia	1–2	1:1	10	16	—
Scoliosis ('idiopathic, adolescent')	0·22	1:6	7	5	—
Spina bifida	0·30	2:3	5[a]	4[a]	—
Tracheo-oesophageal fistula	0·03	1:1	1	1	—

[a] Risk for anencephaly or spina bifida
[b] Additional 1–2% risk of other neural tube defects
[c] If associated with ataxia, or symmetrical spastic paraplegia or athetosis risk approximately 10%

Index

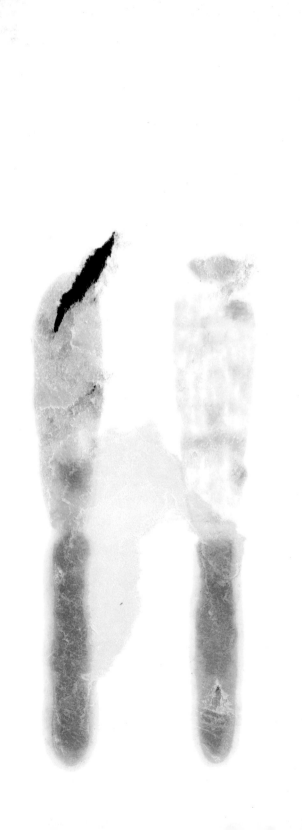

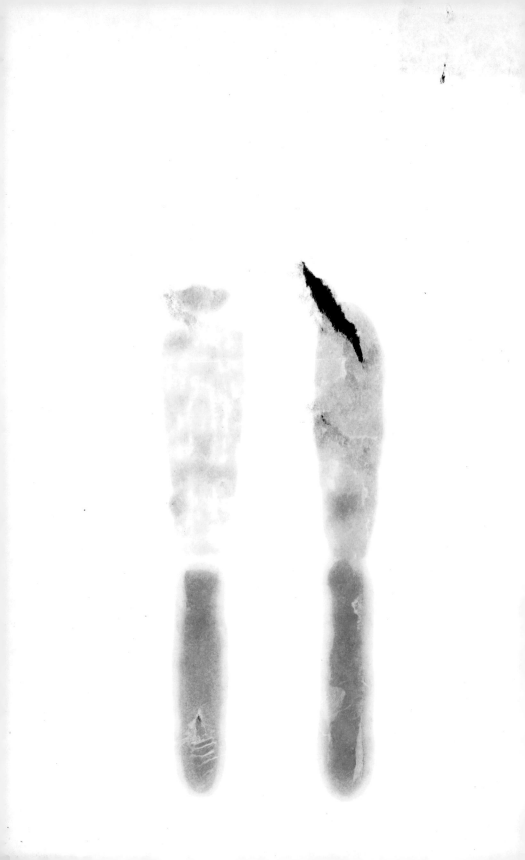